IS OUR FOOD SAFE?

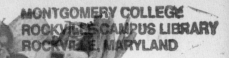

IS OUR FOOD SAFE?

A Consumer's Guide
to Protecting Your
Health and the
Environment

**Warren Leon and
Caroline Smith DeWaal**

Foreword by Michael F. Jacobson

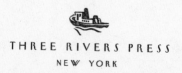

THREE RIVERS PRESS

NEW YORK

Published by Three Rivers Press, New York, New York.
Member of the Crown Publishing Group, a division of Random House, Inc.
www.randomhouse.com

THREE RIVERS PRESS and the Tugboat design are registered trademarks
of Random House, Inc.

Printed in the United States of America

Design by Robert Bull Design

Library of Congress Cataloging-in-Publication Data
Leon, Warren.
    Is our food safe? : a consumer's guide to protecting your health and the
environment / by Warren Leon and Caroline Smith DeWaal.—1st ed.
        p.   cm.
    1. Nutritionally induced diseases—Prevention.   2. Food contamination—
Health aspects.   3. Nutrition.   4. Environmental health.   I. DeWaal,
Caroline Smith.   II. Title.
RC622 .L46 2002
613.2—dc21   2002024146

ISBN 0-609-80782-X

10 9 8 7 6 5 4 3 2 1

First Edition

To my father, Bernard Leon (1923–1995),
who taught me the importance of good health, laughter, and love.
—WL

To my father, Durwood J. Smith, M.D. (1917–1975),
my first and best science teacher.
—CSD

ACKNOWLEDGMENTS

While researching and writing this book, we were helped by many generous, smart people.

Our agent, Faith Hamlin, dispensed ideal doses of sound advice, warm friendship, and no-nonsense information. Shaye Areheart, our editor, suggested we write this book and helped to shape it in crucial ways. Without Faith's and Shaye's unwavering belief in the book, we would not have written it.

Staff members at the Center for Science in the Public Interest (CSPI) provided us with assistance, information, and encouragement. Executive Director Michael Jacobson was especially supportive and allowed us to adapt and expand upon his pamphlet *Nine Weeks to a Perfect Diet* in chapter 5. Bonnie Liebman and Jayne Hurley permitted us to use information from their pamphlet *Healthy Foods: Your Guide to the Best Basic Foods* in that same chapter. Throughout the book, we drew on many of the excellent articles in CSPI's newsletter, *Nutrition Action Healthletter*. Gregory Jaffe, Doug Gurian-Sherman, and David Schardt read sections of the manuscript and provided us with useful advice. In addition, the staff of CSPI's food-safety project, including Leora Vegosen, Kristina Barlow, Arturo (Torey) Riviera, Sara Knavel, Jeremy Wilson, Mina Handa, and Charlotte Christin, provided significant researching and editorial assistance.

Beyond CSPI, Helen Costello and Jeremy Robinson-Leon provided essential research assistance. Helen also wrote several of the profiles. Katherine DiMatteo, Ned Groth, Karen Heisler, John Katz, James Liebman, Margaret Mellon, Richard Wiles, Lori Ann Thrupp, and Kim Waddell shared their knowledge of food issues and pointed us to useful research materials.

With Warren Leon, Michael Brower in 1999 wrote *The Consumer's Guide to Effective Environmental Choices*. We thank Michael for allowing us to use that book's quantitative analysis as the starting point for the discussion of environmental impacts in chapter 3.

We were fortunate that many expert scholars and talented writers were willing to review parts of the manuscript—Michael Brower, Ned Groth, Sallie W. Chisholm, John Katz, Cynthia Robinson, Carl Safina, Debra Simes, and Kaye Wachsmuth. They not only saved us from errors of fact and interpretation, but helped smooth out the rough spots in our writing. Any that remain reflect our stubbornness.

Director of publicity Brian Belfiglio, publicist Tim Roethgen, assistant editor Teryn Johnson, senior production editor Sibylle Kazeroid, copy editor Jim Gullickson, designer Robert Bull, and production manager John Sharp made the process of bringing this book to publication a smooth one and helped us to improve the final product.

The families who have watched their loved ones suffer and sometimes die from something they ate have always provided leadership and inspiration in the fight for a safer food supply. We want to point out the especially important roles of Roni Rudolph, Vicki Peal, Mary Heersink, Laurie Girand, Nancy Donley, and all the families of Safe Tables Our Priority (S.T.O.P.).

We are especially grateful to our own supportive families—Ian, Sophie, and Ethan Smith DeWaal, and Cynthia Robinson and Jeremy Robinson-Leon. They didn't complain about the long hours we spent working on the book. They patiently listened when our findings spilled over into dinnertime conversation. And they accepted changes to their eating patterns as we learned more about which foods protect our health and the environment.

CONTENTS

FOREWORD

The question "Is our food safe?" could not be more timely. The Centers for Disease Control and Prevention estimates that 76 million people get sick, 325,000 are hospitalized, and 5,000 die from contaminated food each year. Poor nutrition, together with a sedentary lifestyle, contributes to heart disease, stroke, cancer, and diabetes—which kill about 400,000 people annually—as well as obesity and other health and dental problems. Chemicals in the food supply may cause cancer, infertility, and changes in fetal development. And now we have the added concern about terrorists intentionally poisoning fresh or processed foods with bacteria or toxic chemicals.

As our food supply increases in complexity and arrives from every corner of the world, consumers get a lot of conflicting advice about what is good to eat and why. Eating more seafood has many nutritional benefits but could result in entire seafood species disappearing from the oceans. Food that is grown with little or no pesticides could still harbor natural hazards. Access to fresh fruits and vegetables year-round is a boon to good nutrition, but not if the foods are contaminated with bacteria or parasites that can make you sick.

In addition, today's consumer is concerned about new hazards like "mad cow disease," which can spread from the meat of infected cattle to humans. Ingredients made from genetically engineered crops are present in countless processed foods. Consumers, who receive propaganda from advocates and opponents, want to know whether they are safe. Moreover, people who have been choosing a more plant-based diet have been distressed to discover that dangerous germs from meat and poultry production can spread to fruits and vegetables both in the field and in the kitchen. Almost daily, news reports on food-poisoning outbreaks, as well as studies from research laboratories, give us insight into what can go wrong with food safety and nutrition.

Meanwhile, advances in food technology can reduce food-safety risks and improve nutrition, but only to the extent that consumers are willing to use them. Irradiation can destroy harmful bacteria in food, but can it also create toxins? Many plants that are genetically modified in a laboratory can be grown with fewer pesticides, but are such foods safe for consumers and the ecosystem?

With so many choices at the grocery stores, it's nearly impossible to know whether a specific food is good for us or for the environment. *Is Our Food Safe?* provides consumers with the up-to-date information they need to answer today's complicated questions about their food choices. With that information, consumers can make choices that will improve both their health and the world we all live in.

This book addresses the broad range of issues needed to make wise food choices, from harmful bugs to helpful labeling. It provides tools for consumers to make their own decisions about what is most important in selecting foods that will prevent foodborne illnesses, improve nutrition, minimize exposure to dangerous chemicals, and protect environmental quality. It also gives specific advice about handling high-risk foods, such as eggs and meat, in the kitchen.

Is Our Food Safe? recognizes that people are not just consumers, but also citizens. Thus, this book gives readers the legal and political background on food-safety controversies. It describes some of the forces—from consumer groups to meat processors—that determine whether our food supply will improve or become more dangerous. Also, it suggests ways in which every reader can help improve the food supply, from getting safer and more nutritious food into your local elementary school to influencing the Congress of the United States. Thus, *Is Our Food Safe?* will empower you to make a difference, not only in your own life, but in the lives of future generations.

Michael F. Jacobson, Ph.D.
Executive Director
Center for Science in the Public Interest

PREFACE

Not too long ago, when people wanted to read about food, they turned to restaurant reviews or recipes in the lifestyle section of their local newspaper. But in recent years, headlines about food safety and the environmental impact of food have been plastered across the front page. Virtually every month there seems to be something new to worry about—mad cow disease, genetically engineered corn, foot-and-mouth disease, water pollution from hog waste, endangered swordfish, *Escherichia coli,* olestra, or *trans* fat.

Although the list of food-related problems continues to expand and seems ever more urgent, it can be maddeningly difficult to figure out what to do. News stories and advice books offer confusing and frequently contradictory suggestions. Some tell us to eat more organic vegetables because they don't contain pesticides, while others warn that those foods may cause food poisoning. Popular diet books advocate eating more beef because of its high protein content, even as nutritionists alert us to its role in heart disease and news stories report on people who become violently ill from eating undercooked hamburger. In the same week, we can read about the benefits to our health from eating more seafood but also be warned of continued sharp declines in ocean fish supplies. Biotechnology companies claim that genetic engineering will provide us with wonderfully healthy new foods while activists warn that it will lead to unprecedented environmental destruction.

Virtually every type of food has been called into question and has caused problems somewhere. Midwesterners who eat lake fish ingest dangerous levels of mercury. Some Massachusetts residents had to boil impure drinking water. Belgians got sick from drinking tainted Coca-Cola. Across Britain, dozens of people contracted a deadly brain disorder by eating meat from diseased cattle. Even such seemingly healthy foods as raspberries and organic apple juice have landed Americans in the hospital.

What's going on? Is our food safe? And what should we eat if we want to protect our health and the environment? These are the questions that this book answers by examining three topics that are usually treated in isolation:

1. Food safety and foodborne illnesses

2. The environmental impacts of different food choices

3. Diet and nutrition

Our goal is to give you a single volume with all the information you need to eat safe, healthy foods in a manner that preserves and protects the environment.

Eating is a very personal act in which you put foreign objects into your body. Each day, you are faced with numerous food decisions. We want to help you make choices that will not only be good for you, but will provide you with pleasure. If you're worried that certain foods might make you sick, cause you to develop a life-threatening illness, or unnecessarily pollute the planet, it will be hard to get much enjoyment from eating them. We therefore point out simple precautions you should take when buying or preparing food and identify which foods you should avoid.

But we won't weigh you down with lengthy lists of instructions that would be hard to keep track of and would turn shopping, cooking, and eating into joyless activities. Instead, in each area—food safety, nutrition, and environment—we suggest a few general rules that can guide you to safe, healthy eating. We point out food fears that have been overblown and food decisions that have trivial implications. In other words, we tell you what you don't need to worry about, as well as what you do.

Is Our Food Safe? follows a middle path between two extremes, with much of the food industry at one end and some food activists at the other. The food industry spends billions of dollars each year on advertising aimed at convincing you that their products are completely safe and essential to your happiness. Just imagine what ads for soft drinks, candy, french fries, or hamburgers would look like if they had to include a balanced assessment of health risks and environmental consequences. We want you to understand the implications of choosing different types of food.

But we won't leave you with the impression that most of your food is tainted or that every trip to the food store or visit to a restaurant is a brush with death. Some food activists, seizing on real food-safety problems and unhappy with the growing power of multinational food corporations, paint a picture of a world on the brink of plague, poverty, and environmental catastrophe. We believe that on balance Americans' food has improved over time, even though our society now faces some new, quite troubling safety and health concerns. Our society's challenge is to fix the problems while preserving the benefits of our current food system.

This book provides commonsense advice that most Americans can follow with relatively little inconvenience or sacrifice. Because we only recommend those actions that are necessary to make the food system safer, we don't ask you to do things that may appeal to those seeking absolute purity but aren't necessary. For example, although we encourage you to cut down on meat consumption, we don't try to convince you that it's essential that you become a vegetarian. Similarly, we don't suggest that periodic visits to a seafood restaurant will destroy the environment or that an occasional stop at a fast-food franchise will doom civilization.

Because food plays a central role in all of our lives and should therefore be an inherently interesting subject, we hope you will find reading this book to be enjoyable as well as useful. Along the way we introduce you to some of the fascinating, inspiring people who are working to make our food system safer and better for the environment.

Before starting out on our journey through your myriad food choices, we want to tell you how we will proceed. We begin in chapter 1 by looking at how and why our current food-safety problems developed. We trace the transition from traditional local, small-scale farms to the current globally intertwined food system. We point out how food consumers have benefited from this shift, as well as the system's disadvantages.

Each of the next six chapters explores a particular food concern. We start with the most immediate and obvious safety question: Will we get sick because of what we eat? In fact, because of bacteria and other microorganisms in our food, millions of Americans become sick each year and thousands of them die. Changes in how food is raised and processed have created new risks of foodborne illness. We identify the key precautionary measures you should take when choosing, preparing, and handling food.

Chapter 3 looks at the relationship between food and environmental quality. We examine which types of food—meat, dairy, fruits, vegetables, and the like—are best and worst for the environment. We provide three key recommendations for choosing foods that protect the environment.

High pesticide use over the past century has affected animals and plants, but do pesticide residues on foods also cause cancer and other diseases in humans? Chapter 4 assesses whether pesticides and other chemicals represent a serious food-safety risk and explains what you should do.

Chapter 5 provides brief, simple-to-follow nutrition advice that is not only good for your health but can also help your waistline. It presents 10 steps to a healthy diet.

The next chapter looks at another increasing concern—biotechnology. Despite the need for much stronger government regulation, consumers do not currently need to avoid genetically engineered foods. Nevertheless, we offer suggestions on how you can help ensure that biotechnology becomes a blessing rather than a curse.

Chapter 7 comes back to the environment to clear up the confusion over some common consumer choices. We discuss whether locally grown foods are superior, whether it's better to eat at home or at a restaurant, how to cut down on the environmental impacts of appliance use, and even whether it matters which bags you ask for at the checkout counter.

Although this book emphasizes your choices as food consumers, along the way we point out actions that the government, food companies, and farmers should take to make the food system safer. In chapter 8, we will discuss how you and other citizens can prod them to improve the way food is grown, distributed, and sold in this country.

The final chapter will put together the separate advice on food safety, nutrition, and the environment so that you can see at a glance which choices, by food category, you should give special attention to.

IS OUR FOOD SAFE?

CHAPTER ONE

IF OUR FOOD IS SO SAFE, WHY ARE WE WORRIED?

Confusing messages about food are everywhere. For example, government leaders tell us we have the safest food supply in the world, but they also ask us to memorize complicated food-handling instructions. Are Americans who question the safety of their food being overcautious, or are there really serious problems with what we eat? In short, is food safety a major concern or not?

At first glance, the situation in America today certainly looks good compared to what it was in the past. After all, we could be living in New York City in the decades leading up to the Civil War. Back then, the public water supply smelled from pollutants and anyone who could afford it paid for water trucked in from the countryside. The milk was so contaminated that newspapers accused the dairies of murder. The cows' meager diet of "swill," residue from the city's distilleries, caused the milk to appear a sickly blue that had to be hidden by artificial coloring. It was then delivered unrefrigerated to local neighborhoods in the same wagons that trucked out cow manure.[1]

The bread wasn't much better. Health reformer Sylvester Graham accused commercial bakers of increasing their profits by adding "chalk, pipe clay and plaster of Paris" to their bread to cover up impurities and to make it heavier and whiter.[2]

New York was by no means unique. At every location and every time in history, people have gotten sick from what they ate. Poor food-preservation techniques, inadequate understanding of sanitation, and contaminants in the food supply caused serious illnesses such as cholera and typhoid fever. Even today, 2 million people die each year in developing countries from diarrheal disease, primarily transmitted through food and water.[3]

Most people throughout history have had diets lacking key nutrients. Before the American Revolution, many of the colonists ate an unvarying diet consisting almost exclusively of bread and meat. For most of the year, they ate few, if any, fruits or vegetables. Even today, many poor people around the world subsist primarily on a single food such as rice. From the lack of vitamins and other essentials, they frequently become sick or blind or even die.

So, viewed through the long lens of history, the modern American food system is a marvel of productivity, cleanliness, and safety. For a visitor from an earlier generation, or from many developing countries today, an American supermarket, with its endless aisles of food choices, including fresh fruits and vegetables stacked high year-round, would be a technological wonder as impressive as computers, video cameras, and cell phones.

This abundance has had real health benefits. People grow taller and live longer than ever before, at least in part because they have more plentiful and better food. We know so much more about nutrition than earlier generations, and our food even comes with informative ingredient lists and nutrition labels. We also use more sophisticated methods to prepare and preserve food safely. Farmers and food processors have raised their standards of sanitation. Government regulators take consumer safety more seriously.

Perhaps most impressive of all, it takes remarkably few people to provide us with all this food. In 1900, more than 2 out of 5 Americans lived on farms, since that was the only way in which society could produce sufficient food. Today, only 1 out of each 40 American workers works in agriculture; and because of their remarkable productivity, the rest of us are free to pursue other occupations and live away from the land.

THE DOWNSIDE TO ALL THAT FOOD

Unfortunately, at the same time that we have increased the variety, quantity, and overall safety of our food, we have created new and serious problems that threaten our well-being. Here are three reasons why we should be concerned.

1. Changes to the Food System Have Generated Troubling New Safety Problems

In a quest for greater productivity and lower costs, farms have changed dramatically since World War II. Farmers now produce much of our food on large commercial farming tracts that grow one or just a few crops. The widespread adoption of a single-crop system, the so-called monoculture, was only possible with the use of chemical agents to increase yields and annihilate pests. Farmers began applying large quantities of synthetic chemical pesticides and fertilizers. The amount of pesticides used annually has now grown to well over 1 billion pounds of active ingredients, 10 times more than in 1945.

Many farmers feel they have little choice but to rely on pesticides once they switch to monoculture. In a farming system in which different crops are grown in rotation, many pests, like potato beetles and corn borers, have difficulty gaining a toehold since they thrive on only one type of plant. But once farmers start growing the same crop in the same field year after year, pesticides become necessary to prevent these pests from flourishing.

While pesticides have allowed farmers to at least partially control pests, they have introduced a new hazard into our lives. Farmworkers and others in farm communities have suffered from pesticide poisoning because of direct contact with the chemicals. The rest of the public has ingested pesticide residues on the food they eat. Lakes, rivers, and groundwater have been polluted. As we will see in chapter 4, pesticides have many harmful effects.

Other changes to the food system have introduced other new hazards. In animal agriculture, large food companies and farmers have constructed massive facilities, some with tens of thousands of pigs or hundreds of thousands of chickens. On such factory-style farms, animals spend their entire lives confined indoors. Many routinely receive antibiotics in their feed, not only to improve growth, but to ward off disease in the crowded, dirty conditions. This practice threatens the continued effectiveness of important antibiotic medicines for humans. And in the crowded, stressful conditions of the large animal farms, disease can spread more quickly, in some cases to humans. Once a problem like *Salmonella* in chickens becomes established on a factory farm, it is extremely difficult to root out.

Modern food-processing practices compound the problem of food-borne illness. For example, not that long ago, local butchers and grocery stores still ground beef on site and packaged it for their customers. If an animal had an infection, the problem was serious but contained. But now, the meat of dozens of cows gets mixed together in a central processing facility. If just one of those animals is diseased, it can infect an entire batch of meat going to thousands of consumers in multiple locations.

Food now also increasingly travels to us from around the world. Trade in food commodities is nothing new—nineteenth-century New Englanders ate wheat from Ohio and molasses from the West Indies and drank tea from India—but these days a much smaller share of the average person's food is produced locally. Increased reliance on imported fruits and vegetables injects new safety risks into the mix, since consumers can't be certain of the conditions under which their food was produced.

If you are like most Americans, you eat a significant share of your meals outside your home. While some restaurants utilize state-of-the-art food-safety protocols, others can't even keep their rest rooms clean. The workforce in America's fast-growing food-service industry includes many of the nation's lowest-paid, youngest, and least-educated workers. Due to a lack of proper equipment or training, necessary safety precautions are not always followed. When a cook at home fails to wash food surfaces properly, perhaps three, four, or five household members are affected. But when an individual in a restaurant or another commercial food-service facility does the same thing, hundreds of people can end up ill.

All of these changes over the past 60 years represent serious causes for concern. Moreover, because of global trade in food and the increasing globalization of disease, there is always the threat that a new food-borne illness will spread from one part of the world to the rest, much as AIDS did in the realm of sexually transmitted disease.

Food-safety problems can crop up in unpredictable, seemingly random ways, heightening public concern. Neither smelling, looking at, or even tasting your food will tell you if it is tainted. You can't see the pesticide residues on your fruit or the pathogens in your meat. Because most people have little contact with farms, the entire food-production process seems mysterious and baffling, much more so than for previous generations.

Paul Slovic and other social scientists who study Americans' attitudes toward risk have concluded that people are much more willing to accept risks that they understand and feel they have some control over. Most Americans realize that high-fat, high-salt, high-sugar diets cause many more deaths and more sickness than pesticides or bacterial contamination of food, but these diet choices are subject to greater individual control. With modern nutrition labels, consumers can frequently identify foods with too much fat or sugar, but they can't tell when they are ingesting invisible microorganisms or chemicals that will harm them.[4]

2. Changes to the Food System over the Past 60 Years Have Caused Widespread, Permanent Environmental Damage

The same trends that have introduced new food-safety concerns have damaged the environment, sometimes in irreversible ways. Pesticides harm beneficial insects and other animals. They also pollute water supplies. Large-scale animal farms are another leading cause of water pollution. Moreover, modern industrial-style monoculture agriculture uses extravagant amounts of freshwater, depleting a valuable resource. Topsoil, another valuable natural resource, washes or blows off fields, in part because the farming methods emphasized in the past 60 years haven't made the preservation of topsoil a priority.[5]

In addition, after World War II farmers began spreading large quantities of chemical nitrogen and phosphorus fertilizers on their fields in order to increase yields. Along with improved plant varieties and increased irrigation, the fertilizers worked well at raising the productivity of farmers' fields. Back in 1940, wheat farmers produced only 15 bushels per acre, but now the yields are nearly three times that much.[6] In more traditional farming, because manure and careful crop rotations add nitrogen back into the soil, all those chemical fertilizers aren't necessary. Our heavy reliance on chemical fertilizers adds large quantities of nitrogen to rivers, lakes, and oceans, where it's doing considerable harm to plants and fish.

Before rejecting modern agricultural methods, we need to acknowledge that they have given us abundant food at low economic costs. Americans spend only about 10 percent of their income on food, a remarkably low amount by historical standards. The cost of food has gone up much less than that of many other products over the past several generations. However, we pay for some of the costs of food not at the grocery store or restaurant but through our taxes, when we have to clean up the environment, and through health insurance premiums that cover illness from drinking polluted water or poisoned fish.

Just as humans have wreaked environmental havoc on land, we've done so at sea. In the last few generations, we've developed technologies and fishing practices that have allowed us to ever more ruthlessly and efficiently extract seafood from the oceans. In many places, the fish can't breed fast enough to replace all the ones we're catching and killing, so fish populations are declining. At the same time, the fishing industry has introduced methods that damage the ocean bottom and other aspects of the marine environment. Even fish farming can have serious adverse effects.

In the quest to produce food cheaply, the food industry has developed technologies and food-production strategies that can harm the environment on a scale much greater than ever before. It's not surprising that many people worry about the potential environmental impacts of the next big technological breakthrough, genetically engineered foods.

3. It Has Become Harder to Maintain a Healthy Lifestyle

Weight gain has reached epidemic proportions, putting many people at risk for heart disease, diabetes, and other diseases. According to the National Health and Nutrition Examination Surveys, the percentage of adults who are overweight increased from 25 percent to 35 percent from the 1970s to the 1990s, while the obesity rate among children ages 6 to 11 jumped from 8 percent to 14 percent.[7] Those disturbing trends have continued since then.

On top of that, many Americans are consuming diets that are low in beneficial foods, such as fruits and vegetables, and are overloaded with those ingredients—fats, sugar, salt—most likely to cause health problems. That is happening even as the average American's knowledge of nutrition has increased and helpful information, especially via nutrition labels on foods, has become more available.

Most Americans would like to eat healthful foods and be physically fit, but it has become harder and harder to do that. Fewer people have jobs that include extensive physical activity, so exercise needs to be incorporated into our leisure hours. But with so many competing pressures on our time, it's hard to fit in adequate exercise. Reliance on cars and the growing popularity of sedentary pastimes only exacerbate the problem.

Almost every hour of the day we receive messages to eat more. Supermarkets have been scientifically designed and carefully arranged to tempt us to increase our food purchases. Elsewhere, we are surrounded by advertisements, billboards, vending machines, and food displays. The food industry bombards us with $25 *billion* worth of advertising and promotions, such as coupons, gift giveaways, and samples. In contrast, the National Cancer Institute spends only $1.4 *million* annually to promote a healthful diet through the "5 a Day" program.[8]

The industries that produce the foods that are worst for us—including snacks, fast foods, sugar beverages, and meat—have especially increased their promotional efforts. Between 1988 and 1999, the number of dollars spent for soft drink advertising rose by 28 percent, for candy and snacks by 40 percent, and for restaurants by 86 percent.[9] Food companies have placed snack products in many new venues to tempt us. We can't walk into a gas station or a pharmacy, or go through a supermarket or a hardware store checkout, without being surrounded by candy bars and potato chips. Vending machines with snack foods and soft drinks accost us in hotel hallways, at highway rest areas, and on subway platforms. As a Coca-Cola executive boasted, "[To] build pervasiveness of our products, we're putting ice-cold Coca-Cola classic and our other brands within reach, wherever you look: at the supermarket, the video store, the soccer field, the gas station—everywhere."[10]

Our schools have unconsciously started to train our children in bad nutrition. Soft drink and snack machines have invaded school hallways, and advertising has entered the classroom through educational-television ventures like Channel One news.

With our mobile, on-the-go lifestyles, Americans are more frequently eating away from home. On average, we now consume one-third of our calories outside the home.[11] But it can be hard to find healthy food choices at restaurants, fast-food franchises, and take-out stands, which mostly feature high-fat, high-salt, high-sugar foods. We are much less likely to eat fruits and healthy vegetables there. For example, we eat more than one-third of our meat and more than two-thirds of our french fries away from home, but less than 10 percent of our fruit.[12] In addition, large food portions and appeals to order appetizers and desserts encourage us to overeat.

These days, it takes careful planning and great willpower to eat a healthy diet. It's not surprising that many people fall short. So, despite our knowledge and desire to be healthy, we Americans increasingly risk disease because of what we eat.

KEEPING THE BABY BUT NOT THE BATHWATER

How should we address these serious problems with the food system? It clearly wouldn't make sense to try to return to an earlier era. Very few of us would find that agreeable. Reducing farm productivity would create scarcity and swell the ranks of the hungry and malnourished.

Few people would be willing to renounce all modern prepared and packaged foods, thereby committing themselves to cooking almost all meals from scratch. Nor would most people be happy if they had to restrict themselves to foods grown in their own locality and region. Those of us in the Northeast or the Midwest would have to give up oranges from Florida, broccoli from California, and bananas from Central America, not to mention more exotic fare like noodles from Japan, olives from Greece, and pineapples from Hawaii. But without taking such radical steps, there is still a lot we can do to ensure our food is good for us and for the environment.

We can appreciate what's good about contemporary food while at the same time encouraging changes in the food system. We can have what's good about it while dramatically reducing the risks to our health and to the environment from current food practices. We can continue to enjoy the variety and convenience that so many appreciate. Farms can continue to be highly productive. Food can remain relatively inexpensive (although perhaps not quite as cheap if we invest more in food safety and environmental protection). Perhaps most important, our food could be much safer and healthier for us while also being at least as tasty and as enjoyable to eat. We can have a food system that provides safer, more nutritious food and improves the environment.

Your individual actions can make a big difference—not only to protect your own health, but to help point the entire food system in the right direction. Your choices and your role are what the rest of this book is about.

CHAPTER TWO

BUGS, MORE BUGS, AND SUPERBUGS: HANDLING HAZARDS IN OUR FOOD

In 1993, the American public woke up to the startling fact that the food supply was not nearly as safe as they had assumed. A major food-poisoning outbreak in the Pacific Northwest was linked to fast-food hamburgers. In the end, over 700 consumers became ill and 4 children died from this food that is synonymous with American culture.[1] The outbreak provided a wake-up call to government leaders, demonstrating that festering problems in the food supply were having a serious impact on the public's health.

Lauren Rudolph was almost seven, with red silky hair and a great smile. She was the first to die (the "sentinel case") in this outbreak, which centered on the Jack in the Box food chain. Right before Christmas 1992, Lauren's father took Lauren and her brother to a Jack in the Box near their home in San Diego to celebrate the children's good grades at school. What Lauren's father didn't know was that the meal contained a deadly bacterium called *Escherichia coli* O157:H7.[2]

E. coli is a common bacterial species that resides in the intestines of both humans and animals. Most strains are completely harmless. However, somewhere in the world, *E. coli* formed a deadly union with a toxin that causes a disease much like dysentery, a condition dreaded in developing countries. The result, *E. coli* O157:H7, is a human pathogen that can live quite happily and harmlessly in the gut of a cow, but once it gets into a human, it can chew up the intestine, causing bloody diarrhea and painful abdominal cramps. The infection can progress to hemolytic-uremic syndrome (HUS) or thrombotic thrombocytopenic purpura (TTP), and can ultimately lead to kidney failure. Although many consumers have immune systems strong enough to fight the toxins, children frequently do not. For that reason, children and adults with weak immune systems (including many elderly consumers) must not be exposed to *E. coli* O157:H7.[3] That is what we know now. But few people knew it when Lauren ate the Jack in the Box hamburger.

On Christmas Eve, Lauren was admitted to the San Diego Children's Hospital following two days of bloody diarrhea. On the day after Christmas, Lauren suffered the first of two massive heart attacks. By then, Roni Rudolph, Lauren's mother, recalls, "Lauren was on a life-support system, her organs shutting down and her kidneys ceasing to function. Her brain waves were almost completely flat. The only movement from her tortured little body was a fluttering of her eyelids every so often caused by a muscle spasm." Two days later, Lauren died following her second heart attack.[4]

That shocking event was only the beginning. Because of an antiquated public health system, for three more weeks the Jack in the Box chain unknowingly continued to sell hamburgers that contained the deadly bacteria. The outbreak spread to three more states. Finally, when very sick children in Seattle, Washington, were overwhelming emergency rooms, public health investigators in Washington State figured out that many of the children had eaten at Jack in the Box. They announced that deadly foodborne illnesses had been linked to the fast-food chain, which suspended operations in Seattle, and the outbreak stopped.[5]

Bert Bartleson, a technical expert for the Washington State Department of Health, who played a critical role in identifying Jack in the Box as the source of the hamburgers and in stopping the outbreak, said:

> While the Jack in the Box outbreak was a victory for the tools of shoe-leather epidemiology, it also showed the glaring weaknesses in the existing public health system. It was difficult to identify large multistate outbreaks of *E. coli* O157:H7 when many of the states did not require reporting. The meat industry at that time did not believe eliminating *E. coli* O157:H7 from ground beef was something they needed to do. In addition, most health departments did not even realize that thin beef patties were often undercooked, since they lacked the tools to accurately measure cooking temperatures. Things had to improve after that.[6]

Roni Rudolph came to Washington, D.C., in 1993 with many other parents whose children had suffered or died in the Jack in the Box outbreak to ask the federal government to close the food-safety gaps that had contributed to Lauren's death. "I cannot help thinking that had the problem [of contaminated meat] been detected earlier; had laws already been in place requiring reporting of *E. coli* O157:H7 cases by physicians and laboratories to local health departments; had laws with strict enforcement already existed for ground meat cooking temperatures; had the USDA required zero tolerance for food contamination; had someone, anyone, cared enough to make sure that our children don't eat hamburgers contaminated with deadly bacteria," Lauren would still be alive, Rudolph told Congress in 1993.[7]

E. coli O157:H7 and other natural hazards in the food supply, including bacteria, parasites, and viruses, are a good reminder of the interconnections between the natural world operating at a microscopic level and our day-to-day lives. Microscopic hazards live in the environment where food is produced and processed. Consumers shouldn't be troubled to learn that bacteria and viruses can live in our food. Bacteria are all around us and most are perfectly safe for consumption. In fact, some types are even beneficial.[8] But others are pathogenic, which means that they can cause illness, or even death.

While people have been coexisting with bacteria since the dawn of time, in recent years both human and bacterial populations have changed. We enjoy advances in medicine that have extended our lives but have affected our immune system. As we age, we grow more susceptible to bacteria in the environment. In addition, these living organisms are continually evolving to adapt to their environment. This can make the harmful ones tough to beat.

Bacteria and other natural hazards pose the largest foodborne risk to the public's health. The Centers for Disease Control and Prevention (CDC) estimates that as many as 76 million people become ill, 325,000 are hospitalized, and 5,000 die in the United States each year from contaminated food.[9] And anyone who has ever been sick with food poisoning knows that the pain can be excruciating, even if it doesn't require hospitalization.

Food poisoning frequently masquerades as a "stomach flu" or a "24-hour bug." Symptoms range from the classic D-N-Vs (which means "diarrhea-nausea-vomiting") to acute life-threatening conditions, like HUS and Guillain-Barré syndrome, to chronic conditions, like reactive arthritis.[10] Illness can occur within a few hours, a few days, or even a few weeks of eating contaminated food, depending on the type of hazard involved. For example, some hazards, like hepatitis A, don't produce illness for many weeks, making it nearly impossible to identify the food source. (See Figure 1.)

The odds of food poisoning's happening to you are very high: 1 out of 4 people will get food poisoning each year. The rates of hospitalization and death from contaminated food are unacceptably high as well. One American in 840 will be hospitalized and 1 in 55,000 will die from contaminated food. The odds are even worse for elderly consumers, children, or those who are immune-compromised.

The food industry can reduce the risk to consumers by reducing the amount of contaminated food that reaches consumers' hands. Consumers can improve their own odds by washing their hands frequently, using safe food-handling practices, cooking their meat thoroughly, and watching for food-recall alerts. Ultimately, both groups play critical roles in ensuring the safety of food.

Highly processed foods, such as canned foods, can be among the safest on the market. But no one wants to exist on a diet consisting principally of canned and prepackaged food, especially since such items come packed with high levels of fat, sugar, or salt. The foods most likely to cause a food-poisoning outbreak are less processed, such as meat, poultry, seafood, eggs, fruits, vegetables, and dairy products.[11]

Food safety can pose a challenge for those who value foods that are minimally processed, such as unpasteurized apple cider. One 1996 outbreak was linked to a well-known juice manufacturer in California called Odwalla, which specialized in producing unpasteurized juice mixes. Over 70 people became ill and 1 child died from the simple act of drinking an Odwalla juice drink made with unpasteurized apple juice. Laurie Girand, the mother of a three-year-old girl named Anna who was hospitalized during that outbreak, said, "When we bought Odwalla juice for Anna, we thought she was getting something that was more healthy for her, never dreaming that it was a drink that had the potential to kill her." While Anna survived her exposure to the deadly *E. coli* that was in the unpasteurized juice, another little girl in Colorado did not.[12] Today, Odwalla juices are flash pasteurized to eliminate *E. coli* and other hazards.

FIGURE 1
MEET THE BUGS

Name	Possible symptoms (from most to least common)	Foods that have been linked to outbreaks	Onset	Duration
Campylobacter	Diarrhea (can be bloody), fever, abdominal pain, nausea, headache, muscle pain	Chicken, raw milk, unchlorinated water	2 to 5 days	7 to 10 days
Ciguatoxin	Numbness, tingling, nausea, vomiting, diarrhea, muscle pain, headache, temperature reversal (hot things cold and cold things hot), dizziness, muscular weakness, irregular heartbeat	Grouper, barracuda, snapper, amberjack, reef fish	Within 6 hours	Several days (neurological symptoms can last weeks or months)
Clostridium botulinum	Marked fatigue; weakness; dizziness; double vision; difficulty speaking, swallowing, and breathing; abdominal distention	Home-canned foods, sausages, meat products, commercially canned vegetables, seafood products, garlic in oil	18 to 36 hours	Fatal in 3 to 10 days if not treated
Cyclospora (parasite)	Watery diarrhea, loss of appetite, weight loss, cramps, nausea, vomiting, muscle aches, low-grade fever, extreme fatigue	Raspberries, lettuce, basil	1 week	Ranges from a few days to 30 days or more
E. coli O157:H7	Severe abdominal pain, watery (then bloody) diarrhea, occasionally vomiting. Can lead to hemolytic-uremic syndrome (HUS) in children, which causes acute kidney failure. A similar illness, thrombotic thrombocytopenic purpura (TTP), may occur in adults.	Ground beef, raw milk, lettuce, sprouts, unpasteurized juices	1 to 8 days	Abdominal pain, diarrhea, and vomiting last about 8 days. HUS and TTP can cause death.

Name	Possible symptoms (from most to least common)	Foods that have been linked to outbreaks	Onset	Duration
Hepatitis A (virus)	Fever, malaise, nausea, loss of appetite, abdominal pain, jaundice	Shellfish, salads, cold cuts, sandwiches, fruits, vegetables, fruit juices, milk, dairy products, infected handlers	10 to 50 days	1 to 2 weeks
Listeria monocytogenes	Fever, chills, headache, nausea, vomiting, diarrhea, infection of the blood (septicemia), inflammation of the membranes of the brain or spinal cord (meningitis), spontaneous abortion or stillbirth	Hot dogs, deli meats, raw meat, poultry, raw vegetables, smoked fish, raw milk, soft cheeses such as Camembert and queso blanco, ice cream	A few days to 3 weeks	Variable; can be fatal if not treated
Norwalk (virus)	Nausea, vomiting, diarrhea, abdominal pain, headache, fever	Shellfish, salads, infected food handlers	1 to 2 days	1 to 2½ days
Salmonella	Nausea, vomiting, abdominal cramps, diarrhea, fever, headache	Poultry, eggs, raw meats, dairy products, fish, cream-filled desserts, produce	6 hours to 2 days	1 to 2 days
Scombrotoxin	Tingling or burning sensation in the mouth, upper-body rash, reduced blood pressure, headache, itching, nausea, vomiting, diarrhea	Fresh tuna, mahimahi, bluefish, sardines, mackerel, amberjack	Immediate to 30 minutes	3 hours to several days
Vibrio parahaemoly ticus	Diarrhea, abdominal pain, nausea, vomiting, headache, fever, chills	Raw oysters, clams, mussels, crabs, shrimp	4 hours to 4 days	2½ days
Vibrio vulnificus	Diarrhea (in healthy people); bloodstream infection (in people with liver disease, diabetes, or a weak immune system)	Raw oysters, clams, mussels	Within 16 hours (diarrhea)	2–8 days; can be fatal in people with liver disease, diabetes, or a weak immune system

The initial government response to this outbreak was to propose mandatory pasteurization for all juices. Many consumer advocates balked at the idea that "fresh," minimally processed juices should be banned and, instead, supported more modest reforms. Unfortunately, the outbreaks from unpasteurized juices have continued, and it is clear that the only short-term solution to protect children like Anna is to require that all juices be pasteurized or otherwise treated to eliminate harmful bacteria.

Assuring safety while preserving our ability to enjoy food that is minimally processed can present difficult choices for consumers who value both.

This chapter will cover the types of natural hazards that show up in different foods, from the well-known to the unexpected. Using information and analysis from food-poisoning outbreaks (where two or more people become ill from a specific contaminated food), it describes what risks to anticipate and what you can do to prevent food poisoning. Unfortunately, not all hazards can be prevented by the consumer, and these must be controlled earlier in the food chain. But consumers can do a lot to reduce their risk, especially from raw animal products like meat, poultry, seafood, and eggs. These pose the greatest risk of causing illness, either from undercooking or from improper handling in the kitchen that spreads bacteria to uncooked food items.

FOUR STEPS TO AVOID FOOD POISONING

- Beware the bugs that can spread around your kitchen, from hand to plate, from meat to salad. Wash hands, counters, plates, and utensils frequently, especially after contact with raw meats or eggs.

- Wash fresh produce under running water to dislodge bacteria.

- Thoroughly cook meat, poultry, fish, and eggs.

- Practice 2 hours/2 inches/4 days for leftovers: two hours maximum to leave leftovers out of the refrigerator, two inches thick to cool leftovers quick, and four days in the refrigerator.

FIGURE 2
MEAT AND POULTRY OUTBREAKS, 1990–2001

Total number of reported outbreaks linked to meat: 273

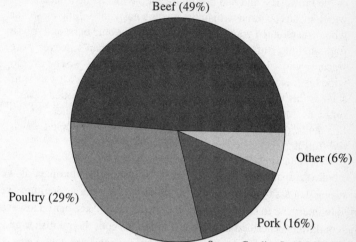

Source: Caroline Smith DeWaal et al.,
Outbreak Alert!: Closing the Gaps in Our Federal Food Safety Net, rev. ed.
(Washington, D.C.: Center for Science in the Public Interest, 2001), p. 10.

MEAT AND POULTRY

Lauren Rudolph and her family are not the only victims of an antiquated system of producing and inspecting meat and poultry. Millions of people become sick each year from hazards commonly found on meat or poultry products, according to the U.S. Department of Agriculture. Those hazards exist despite the fact that the federal government employs over 7,500 inspectors who visit meat and poultry plants at least once each day. These products are "inspected" more than any other foods, but the inspection techniques were largely devised nearly 100 years ago to address animal diseases that could spread to humans.[13]

Today's food-safety system was adopted by Congress in 1906 in response to publication of *The Jungle,* the best-selling novel by Upton Sinclair. His fictionalized investigative report exposed conditions in the

Chicago stockyards and stimulated a powerful public reaction. In one particularly disturbing passage, Sinclair wrote:

> There were cattle which had been fed on "whiskey-malt," the refuse of the breweries, and had become what the men called "steerly"— which means covered with boils. It was a nasty job killing these, for when you plunged your knife into them they would burst and splash foul-smelling stuff into your face; and when a man's sleeves were smeared with blood and his hands steeped in it, how was he ever to wipe his face, or to clear his eyes so that he could see? It was stuff such as this that made the "embalmed beef" that had killed several times as many United States soldiers as all the bullets of the Spaniards; only the army beef, besides, was not fresh canned, it was old stuff that had been lying for years in the cellars.[14]

Not surprisingly, the book generated considerable outrage, as well as strong denials by the meat industry. The secretary of agriculture even tried to intervene to stop distribution of the book by U.S. mail. However, the conditions described in it were verified by both the publisher and a separate government commission. Consumers demanded a response.

While Congress had been considering legislation to clean up conditions in the meatpacking industry for years, publication of *The Jungle* provided the impetus to move the bills through Congress. Within six months of the book's publication, Congress passed both the Pure Food Act and the Meat Inspection Act. These laws continue to provide the foundation of food-safety regulation in the United States today.

In the 1990s, when the Jack in the Box outbreak occurred, meat inspection was largely unchanged from the system adopted in 1906. By 1995, the Clinton administration recognized the importance of addressing the problem of unsafe meat. Proposals were written, battles were fought in Congress, and finally, in July 1996, President Clinton announced a new regulation to modernize meat and poultry inspection that required the food industry to control food-safety hazards, like the one that killed Lauren, using a system called HACCP (Hazard Analysis and Critical Control Points).[15] The meat industry's HACCP plans were monitored by the government, under a system that included both inspection and microbiological testing. This was the first time that laboratory testing of meat products was ever done as part of a government regulatory program. That change has been highly successful—for example, resulting in reductions of one hazard, *Salmonella,* in meat products by one-third to one-half in just two years.[16] It would have been nice if this had been the end of the story, but unfortunately it wasn't.

In January 1999, another food-poisoning outbreak captured the nation's attention. A well-known food processor, Sara Lee, produced luncheon meats and hot dogs that sickened 100 people and killed 21.[17] Its cause? Another deadly bacterium, *Listeria monocytogenes,* which is found in a wide variety of ready-to-eat foods, including hot dogs, luncheon meat, soft cheese, smoked fish, and deli salads.

This bacterium has two daunting characteristics that make it very challenging for the food industry. First, unlike most bacteria, *Listeria* can grow in the refrigerator. Many food hazards are controlled simply by keeping food cold. But *Listeria* is different: low contamination levels in a ready-to-eat food can reach hazardous levels even when the food is refrigerated.[18]

Second, *Listeria monocytogenes* is frequently fatal. While most of us have immune systems that will kill it off before it has a chance to make us sick, *Listeria* poses a serious hazard for a growing number of consumers, including pregnant women and the elderly. In addition, the cases of illness are particularly severe. Nine out of 10 people who become ill are hospitalized, with hospital stays averaging two weeks. And 20 to 40 percent of those who become ill will die.[19] Frequently, those deaths are miscarriages, because pregnant women can pass the hazard to their fetuses. *Listeria*'s high death rate is second only to that of *Vibrio vulnificus,* a hazard found in shellfish. Taken together, these factors mean that food processors must keep *Listeria* out of their products.

Although the government banned ready-to-eat foods that contain hazardous types of *Listeria* in the late 1980s, that prohibition is enforced using a weak government program that only rarely tests food already in the marketplace. The government has never required food processors to check their products and plants to ensure that they are controlling *Listeria* before they send the food to consumers.[20] The Sara Lee outbreak clearly demonstrated that more effective monitoring and testing for foodborne hazards is needed in order to protect the public from these deadly pathogens.

Clearly, the Clinton administration's efforts to improve meat and poultry safety provided only a partial solution. The food industry and the government must keep a vigilant watch for emerging food-safety hazards, such as antibiotic-resistant bacteria and mad cow disease, while at the same time maintaining and improving protections against old hazards, like *E. coli* O157:H7 and deadly strains of *Listeria*. Consumers can monitor developments in the media while keeping bacteria from spreading in their kitchens.

Luckily, many food-safety hazards associated with meat and poultry products can be almost completely eliminated with proper handling and thorough cooking. With better understanding of the hazards and care in the kitchen, consumers can prevent many illnesses.

The bacteria that can make you sick frequently aren't the same as the bacteria that cause food to spoil. Therefore, illness-causing bacteria can be present on food that doesn't smell, taste, or look odd or spoiled. Most bacteria will not grow if the food is held at refrigerated temperatures below 40 degrees Fahrenheit. (*Listeria* is an exception.) But they can grow rapidly in foods held between 40 and 140 degrees—the "danger zone."[21]

In handling raw meat or poultry, always assume that it harbors harmful bacteria. Before preparing meat products, clear the counter and thoroughly clean it. Clean everything, including sponges and hands, that comes in contact with the raw meat or its juice immediately with hot, soapy water.[22] Sanitize sponges by running them through your dishwasher or "cooking" them in your microwave.

Meat and poultry should always be defrosted and marinated in the refrigerator, not on the counter. At room temperature, bacteria that are present on the meat surface will have a chance to grow, even if the meat is still frozen on the inside. Thawing food in the refrigerator takes a little extra time, but doing so is critical to ensure that the bacteria stay at low levels on the surface of the meat, reducing the likelihood of cross-contamination in the kitchen or cooking errors. A microwave will also defrost food safely and quickly.

Marinade used for raw meat should be gently heated (to 160 degrees) before it is used to baste meat or for gravy. Otherwise, you are simply reapplying bacteria from the raw to the cooked meat.

Ground-meat products are especially hazardous, because they are made from both the exterior (which harbors bacteria) and the interior of the meat, spreading bacteria throughout the mix. Hamburgers and ground poultry must be cooked to 160 degrees all the way through to eliminate the risk from *E. coli* O157:H7 and other harmful bacteria. Rare and medium-rare hamburgers are too risky to eat these days, unless you are using irradiated ground beef.

The USDA recommends that all consumers (even backyard barbecuers) use a thermometer when cooking ground meat to ensure that the center has reached 160 degrees.[23] Gently insert the thermometer so that it penetrates only halfway through. Disposable thermometers and instant-read thermometers are making this easier than ever.

For intact cuts of meat, like steaks and roasts, you can cook them to a rare or medium-rare temperature (which is still a little pink in the middle). Once the surface is fully cooked, you have eliminated the hazard. However, if you use a fork to pierce or tenderize the meat, this allows bacteria to enter. Then the meat should be cooked medium or well-done (no pink in the middle) to eliminate the risk.

For poultry, you should also use a meat thermometer. While more and more whole turkeys and chickens come with a pop-up thermometer, it's a good idea to check the temperature with a conventional meat thermometer, such as an oven-safe, dial instant-read, or a digital thermometer.[24] Set the oven no lower than 325 degrees and cook the turkey or chicken to 180 degrees, taking the reading in the thick part of the thigh.

Leaving cooked food at room temperature is an invitation for common bacteria like *Clostridium perfringens* and *Staphylococcus aureus* to grow in your food and produce sickening toxins. If cooked food has been left out for more than two hours, throw it away. Reheating will not destroy the toxin produced by *Staphylococcus aureus* nor the spores of *Clostridium perfringens.* [25]

Food should be chilled as quickly as possible in the refrigerator. For a classic turkey dinner, for example, this means you should divide the turkey into smaller pieces and store the meat separately from the stuffing and the gravy.[26] To drop the temperature fast, store leftovers at a shallow depth—about two inches. Shallow containers allow food to cool more evenly and quickly in the refrigerator or freezer.

More on turkeys: The USDA recommends that stuffing be prepared separately from the turkey.[27] That is because turkey farmers have developed turkeys that actually cook faster, so that your turkey might be done before your stuffing is.

Stuffing is warm and moist—a perfect environment for bacteria to grow. Stuffing can be contaminated by bacteria from eggs and shellfish in the stuffing or from the turkey itself. If you are preparing the stuffing ahead of time, wet and dry ingredients should be refrigerated separately and mixed just before cooking.

For many people, stuffing cooked inside the turkey is one of the best parts of the meal. If you are one of these people, loosely stuff the turkey just before you stick it in the oven with three-fourths of a cup of stuffing per pound of turkey. Use a meat thermometer to make sure the center of the stuffing reaches 165 degrees. If the turkey is done but the stuffing isn't, simply remove the stuffing from the turkey and cook it on the stove before serving it. This dual cooking gives you all the flavor without the risk. Avoid prestuffed fresh turkeys.

Finally, to reduce the risk from *Listeria* in ready-to-eat meats, pregnant women, the elderly, and the immune deficient should avoid patés, uncooked hot dogs, and luncheon meat.

ACTIVISM FOR ALEX

Nancy Donley never wanted to be an activist for consumers. To this day, she wishes she had never needed to become one. Nancy started her journey toward activism in a hospital room as she watched her son lie dying. The death of Alexander Thomas Donley was both a death and a birth for Nancy.

Alex Donley was six years old and Nancy and Tom Donley's only child. His parents were ever mindful of Alex's safety. "Until he was six, I wouldn't even let him in the backyard by himself. In stores, he had to be with me every single second. His seat belt went on automatically," Nancy Donley told *Redbook* magazine in August 2000.

Alex had a heart of gold. He visited with seniors with Parkinson's disease, played with a Down's syndrome student at school, and would always have a hug and a smile for everyone. That all changed after a family cookout in 1993. Alex ate a hamburger that was contaminated with a deadly strain of *E. coli* bacteria.

Alex's horrendous illness lasted four days and ended at Children's Memorial Hospital in Chicago. Alex's kidneys shut down. His brain swelled and a lung collapsed. He developed tremors and stopped recognizing his mother. His eyes stopped focusing. Shortly thereafter, he collapsed into a coma and passed away, following a massive seizure. Doctors diagnosed Alex with HUS, a disease associated with *E. coli*

FOOD SAFETY BEGINS ON THE FARM

There have been many changes in farming that affect food safety. Factory farming has increased dramatically. These farms produce large numbers of animals in confinement systems to minimize costs and shorten the time between birth and slaughter. These farms can become a breeding ground for human pathogens, like *Salmonella* and *Campylobacter*. They also increase the need to treat animals with antibiotics to prevent the development and spread of animal diseases. The pressure to grow animals faster has also led to the recycling of animal by-products into animal feed. The serious—and unexpected—consequences of these changes on the farm are just now becoming apparent.

In 1986, a new disease was identified in British cattle. It was marked by cattle who stumbled and appeared disoriented and aggressive. Nicknamed "mad cow disease," the disease spread to many farms around

O157:H7 infection. More than 70,000 people a year are infected with this virulent strain of bacteria and hundreds die. Children, the elderly, and the chronically ill are the most vulnerable.

Nancy Donley took her grief and turned it into action. She joined with other parents of children who had faced harrowing illnesses and sometimes death because of contaminated food. Together they formed Safe Tables Our Priority (S.T.O.P.), a grassroots organization dedicated to raising awareness, assisting food-poisoning victims, and advocating for stronger government programs to ensure food safety and protect public health. Nancy and the other parents who formed S.T.O.P. have played a critical role in supporting food-safety improvements for the meat and poultry industry. Nancy continues to monitor these improvements as a member of the National Advisory Committee for Meat and Poultry Inspection, appointed by the secretary of agriculture.

"My involvement is in dedication to Alex, who wanted to be a paramedic when he grew up so that 'I can help others,'" Nancy Donley says. "My desire is to live out my life as Alex would have wanted to live out his own, if it hadn't been cut tragically short. I'm attempting in my small way to help others; to be the voice for those forever silenced."*

* Quoted in "100 Women Making a Difference," *Today's Chicago Woman,*
  July 1997.

Great Britain. Mad cow disease has the technical name of bovine spongi-form encephalopathy (BSE). This fatal disease causes the brain to develop lesions and holes. It is untreatable today. BSE is one type of transmissible spongiform encephalopathy, or TSE, a family of diseases that can infect many species, including humans, sheep, mink, and cattle. The disease is believed to be transmitted from a sick individual to a healthy one through consumption of the infected tissue. Human cases were first documented among a New Guinea tribe that practiced cannibalism.[28]

In Britain, mad cow disease reached epidemic proportions in the cattle population before it was recognized to be a human health issue. It was spread because of the practice of feeding cattle the rendered remains of other cattle infected with the disease. While cattle are vegetarians by nature, beef producers introduced the practice of "cannibalism" to fatten cattle quickly in preparation for slaughter. When this practice was first disclosed to the American public, Oprah Winfrey, a popular television talk show host, swore she would never eat another hamburger—and was promptly sued by the cattle industry, which said she was disparaging its product.[29]

Mad cow disease became an international public health concern in 1996 after public health officials in Britain documented that human TSE cases (called a new variant of Creutzfeldt-Jakob disease, or vCJD) were linked to beef consumption, thus showing for the first time that this ter-rible disease could jump the "species barrier" from cattle to humans.[30]

Mad cow disease has become a safety issue for beef consumers all over Europe. Infected cattle have been discovered in many other coun-tries, including France, Portugal, Switzerland, Belgium, Denmark, Liech-tenstein, Luxembourg, the Netherlands, Germany, Spain, and Japan. There are also human cases of vCJD in France. The United States has so far escaped the problem largely because in 1989 the government banned the entry of cattle from countries known to have BSE.[31]

Not unlike what happened in the United States following publica-tion of *The Jungle,* mad cow disease decimated the British beef industry and destroyed faith in that country's system for ensuring food safety. It has shaken European consumers' confidence in government oversight of the food supply. It has led to the revision of food-safety laws and the cre-ation of new agencies that are responsible for ensuring the safety of the food supply, both in Great Britain and other European countries.[32]

ADVICE ON MAD COW DISEASE FOR TRAVELERS

The risk of developing BSE from eating a few servings of beef is minuscule. But if you want to be ultrasafe, here are several tips.

1. The easiest way to avoid BSE in foreign countries is to avoid beef products.

2. If you are going to eat beef, stay away from hamburgers, hot dogs, and sausages, because they are more likely to contain central nervous system (CNS) material, compared with other cuts of beef. (CNS tissue is most likely to carry the infectious agent, known as a prion.)

3. Boneless steaks, roasts, and whole cuts are much safer than T-bones, porterhouses, standing rib roasts, prime ribs with bone, bone-in rib steaks, and bone-in chuck roasts, as the bones may contain spinal-cord tissue.

4. Be careful even outside of Europe. England alone exported tainted meat to over 70 countries. Experts say that the next epidemic of BSE could occur in Russia or Asia.

BSE is just one example of how practices on the farm can affect food safety. Another example is the use of antibiotics in animal production. Antibiotics were first developed for use in human medicine to kill off disease-causing bacteria. Development of the first antibiotic, penicillin, is still considered a medical landmark. With widespread use, however, antibiotics become less effective because bacteria develop tools to resist them. Antibiotics can wipe out most bacteria in a population, but the ones that survive have natural resistance. They reproduce and multiply, and soon the antibiotic has become useless in treating the disease.[33]

In animal production, antibiotics are used not only for the appropriate purpose of treating disease in individual animals. They are routinely, and less appropriately, added to livestock's feed or drinking water to improve growth and feed efficiency. The government does not keep track of antibiotic use, but a recent independent study estimated that 70 percent of antibiotics sold in the United States are fed to livestock, especially

SHOULD FOOD BE IRRADIATED?

Irradiation is a food-processing tool that some companies are using to destroy pathogens on food. Irradiation uses gamma rays, electron beams, and X rays to kill bacteria in foods. It does that effectively, virtually eliminating disease-causing bacteria.

Unfortunately, irradiation is not foolproof. For example, it doesn't kill viruses or prions. There are also foods, like lettuce, that do not weather treatment with irradiation well. Irradiation has a slight effect on the taste of certain foods, and reduces by 10 to 15 percent the levels of certain vitamins. And if the food is highly contaminated, low doses of irradiation might not be totally effective. Therefore, irradiation is not a substitute for good sanitation at food plants.

Some people fear that irradiation will make the food radioactive. That concern is groundless. While irradiation can produce tiny amounts of harmful by-products (similar to those in cooked food), most irradiated food will be safer than traditional food because irradiation kills bacteria and

chickens and pigs, for nontherapeutic uses. Some poultry producers may be cutting back but antibiotic use remains widespread.[34]

This practice has given rise to antibiotic-resistant strains of *Salmonella* and *Campylobacter.* In Europe, for example, antibiotics were given to farm animals so widely and indiscriminately that new bacterial strains—like *Salmonella* Typhimurium DT104—developed that are multidrug resistant. These bacteria can cause human illnesses that resist treatment with up to five different antibiotics.[35] As antibiotic use on the farm has increased, the tools of modern medicine have grown less effective in treating many types of human infections.

In the United States, one such superbug emerged less than five years after the FDA approved the use of an important class of antibiotic—fluoroquinolones—on poultry to prevent flocks from being wiped out from infections caused by *E. coli* and other bacteria. That use was strongly opposed by the Centers for Disease Control and Prevention (CDC), which wrote a letter to the FDA in 1995. The CDC said, "The widespread use of FQs [fluoroquinolones] in animals, even when limited to therapeutic use, will hasten the emergence of resistance, especially in bacteria transmitted by food." Concerns were also strong because the drugs were administered to poultry in drinking water, which raised the

parasites that cause illness. Irradiation has been approved for a variety of foods, including flour, fruits, vegetables, spices, meat, poultry, and eggs.

A 1996 survey conducted for CSPI showed that 92 percent of consumers want irradiated foods to be labeled. Irradiated foods are required by law to bear a symbol called a "radura" on the package and a written description such as "treated by irradiation."

Consumers who are most at risk for contracting foodborne illness, such as elderly, ill, or immunocompromised individuals, may want to purchase irradiated foods. The increased safety factor added by this processing step can decrease the chances of contracting foodborne illness. Nevertheless, despite the hopes of some proponents who view irradiation as a panacea for public concerns about the safety of the food supply, consumer confidence in the safety of food will ultimately depend on making food clean to begin with, not on irradiation as the final processing step. More information about irradiation can be found online at www.cdc.gov/ncidod/dbmd/diseaseinfo/foodirradiation.htm.

issue of environmental release of the antibiotic.[36] The FDA approved fluoroquinolones for use in poultry, despite the opposition. The FDA then documented a marked increase in poultry contaminated with *Campylobacter* that can resist treatment with the new drugs.[37]

Because fluoroquinolones are powerful antibiotics that are important for treating human foodborne infections, *Campylobacter* infections in humans could become harder and harder to treat unless the trend toward resistance is reversed.

In a 1999 CDC study of chicken purchased at retail markets, fluoroquinolone-resistant *Campylobacter* was present in over 10 percent of the samples, and a government risk assessment said that chickens harboring these tough new bacteria could sicken an estimated 11,000 people annually, resulting in prolonged illnesses and complications. On the basis of that evidence, in 2000 the FDA asked companies to stop marketing fluoroquinolones to poultry farmers, a move supported by many in the public health community.[38] However, the leading manufacturer, Bayer, refused to comply with the voluntary withdrawal.

Even though the federal government has begun to take the antibiotic-resistance problem more seriously and has put some useful policies in place, there is little excuse for continuing to allow healthy animals to be routinely fed antibiotics that are important for treating human illness. In the 1990s, the European Union banned the use of a number of antibiotics as growth promoters in animals if the same or similar antibiotics were also used to treat human diseases. That action was vindicated when a study at the Danish Veterinary Laboratory showed that after antibiotics were eliminated from animal feed, the number of antibiotic-resistant microbes dropped dramatically on pigs and chickens. In the case of *Enterococcus faecium* found on chickens, the number resistant to a key antibiotic fell from 73 percent to 6 percent. This is important news since that bug can cause serious infections in hospital patients and could run rampant if no antibiotics were able to treat it.[39]

The World Health Organization (WHO) has called for banning antibiotics in animal feed worldwide, noting that antibiotics have too often become a substitute for high-quality animal hygiene. Livestock do fine without having antibiotics regularly inserted in their food as long as they are "given enough space, clean water and high-grade feed,"[40] according to the WHO report. Of course, when an animal becomes sick, it should be treated with antibiotics if such treatment would cure the illness.

BSE and antibiotic resistance clearly show that practices on the farm have the potential to introduce new hazards into the food supply. Farmers and producers must recognize their critical role in maintaining a safe food supply. Government food-safety programs must begin on the farm to increase their impact.

FRUITS AND VEGETABLES

Many consumers mistakenly believe that they can avoid food-safety problems simply by avoiding foods of animal origin, especially meat and poultry. Although there are significant concerns associated with meat and poultry, fruits and vegetables have their own risks. Harmful bacteria like *E. coli* O157:H7 and *Salmonella* have shown up again and again on fruits and vegetables. Contamination can occur from a variety of sources: irrigation water, direct application of manure, or even dripping fluids from raw meat that get on vegetables in a home or restaurant kitchen.

One 1996 outbreak linked to contaminated lettuce demonstrates how these problems can develop. In all, this lettuce sickened 61 people in three states and hospitalized 21, including 3 children who suffered severe complications. One little girl, three-year-old Haylee Bernstein, spent 14 weeks in the hospital, including 11 weeks in intensive care, fighting the devastating effects of deadly *E. coli* that she ate on fancy premixed lettuce that her mother picked up at a local supermarket.

A *New York Times* investigation of this outbreak concluded that the lettuce producer, Fancy Cutt, took "virtually no measures to protect its salad mixes from contamination." State and federal investigators found the California barn where the contaminated lettuce came from. In it, locally grown greens like radicchio, frisée, and arugula were mixed together in a big stainless-steel tub.

Just outside the barn, cattle—the animal "reservoir" for the deadly *E. coli* bacterium—were kept in a small pen. Bacteria originate in the cattle's manure and from there can contaminate many other foods. According to the *New York Times* report,

> the barn that was Fancy Cutt's processing shed was completely open on one side, exposing the large, stainless steel tub where the leaves of lettuce were washed before being mixed and shipped in three-pound boxes. Less than 100 feet away were some cattle. . . . "Routes of contamination" were all around, wrote an F.D.A. inspector, Mary C. B. Acton. Cow feces could be blown into the shed by wind, washed in by rain and tracked in on worker's boots, by animals or by the birds investigators saw flying into the barn.[41]

The Fancy Cutt outbreak highlights many issues that surround the safety of fresh fruits and vegetables. In the past, produce was grown and consumed locally. A food-safety hazard used to be a local phenomenon, and growers were directly accountable to the public that they supplied, including their family, friends, and neighbors.

Today, advances in transportation and refrigeration have enabled farmers to ship fresh fruits and vegetables not only around the country but around the world. This means that food-safety hazards may show up in states or countries far from where the food was produced. It takes talented detectives at the CDC and state health departments to track food-safety problems to their source. Many outbreaks go unrecognized. Thus, the informal accountability of years past is gone.

FIGURE 3
FRUIT AND VEGETABLE OUTBREAKS, 1990–2001

Total number of reported outbreaks linked to produce: 148

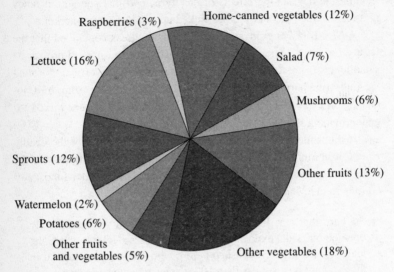

Raspberries (3%)

Home-canned vegetables (12%)

Lettuce (16%)

Salad (7%)

Mushrooms (6%)

Sprouts (12%)

Other fruits (13%)

Watermelon (2%)

Potatoes (6%)

Other fruits and vegetables (5%)

Other vegetables (18%)

Source: Smith DeWaal et al., *Outbreak Alert!*, p. 8.

The Fancy Cutt outbreak is just one example of another worrisome trend. Fruits and vegetables represent a significant cause of food-poisoning outbreaks, including such hazards as parasites imported on Guatemalan raspberries, deadly *E. coli* on lettuce, and *Salmonella* illnesses linked to clover and alfalfa sprouts. In fact, fruits and vegetables are among the top three foods linked to foodborne outbreaks and illness, following seafood and eggs.[42]

In retrospect, this finding is not as surprising as one might think. In both traditional and organic agriculture, animal manure is frequently used as fertilizer or as a soil enhancer. While that practice is valuable, it can also introduce hazards into the environment where food is grown. It is common practice to eat fruits and vegetables raw, with little preparation at home other than washing and chopping. Thus, if a hazard is on the fruit or vegetable when it is purchased by the consumer, it is probably going to be on the food when it is eaten.

The government imposes no restrictions on the use of manure on food crops, although organic food products must meet voluntary new standards for manure use to become certified. That contrasts sharply with the treatment of human sewage; its use on food crops is intensively regulated. Robert Tauxe of the CDC says that a huge leap in public health protection occurred more than 100 years ago when human sewage was removed from the human food supply. The next leap—and our current challenge—is to get animal manure (and related hazards like *Salmonella* and *E. coli* O157:H7) out of the human food supply. However, this must be done with an understanding of farm ecology and the value of manure for soil. Raising healthier animals that carry fewer human pathogens may provide a long-term solution, but, in the near term, farmers should ensure the safe use of manure on lands where food crops are growing. Application of manure three to six months prior to seeding the ground, especially in cold climates, is probably adequate to eliminate the risk.[43] More research is needed on methods of composting and handling manure in order to give better guidance to farmers.

Today, no federal agency has regulatory responsibility over food safety on the farm unless an actual outbreak occurs. Agriculture has been an economic building block of the country, and farmers hold a surprising amount of political power in the nation's capital. Efforts to implement on-farm food-safety standards in the farm belt are met with strong opposition, but, as disease outbreaks amply demonstrate, better controls are urgently needed.

The best advice for consumers is simply to wash fresh fruits and vegetables under running water.[44] Washing produce under running water is more effective than soaking it to remove bacteria and dirt because the pressure of the water can help dislodge contaminants. For hard vegetables, like carrots, use a small scrub brush. Cutting away bruised or damaged areas increases the safety and has the added benefit of making the vegetable more appealing. Sprays and other products for washing fruits and vegetables aid in the removal of wax and dirt, and those could be useful in removing pathogens and pesticides as well.

While these practices will help make your produce safer to eat, washing alone is no guarantee of safety, because there are too many places for bacteria to hide on the rough surface of many fruits and vegetables.

SPROUTS: EAT AT YOUR OWN RISK

Sprouts are a real favorite among health-food connoisseurs, but they have also been implicated in several far-reaching outbreaks. One outbreak that brought the issue of contaminated sprouts to the public's attention occurred in June 1996. Over 600 people became ill and 1 person died in California after eating alfalfa sprouts contaminated with *Salmonella*. Public health officials investigating the outbreak found insanitary conditions at both the farm and production facilities that contributed to the contamination. The farm that supplied the sprouts collected and stored horse manure next to the alfalfa fields and used chicken manure as a fertilizer. In the sprouting-production facility, the floors were dirty, the same buckets were used for finished sprouts and waste, and there was evidence of flies and rodents. In response to this and other outbreaks, the FDA implemented additional controls, but in 1999 former FDA commissioner Jane E. Henney warned: "Despite all these efforts to make raw sprouts safer, we continue to receive reports of illness associated with raw sprouts. Consumers need to understand that at this time, the best way to control this risk is not to eat raw sprouts."

Despite the modest risks, everyone should still eat plenty of fruits and vegetables, which offer a wide range of nutritional benefits. Microbial safety problems are minimal compared to the importance of fruits and vegetables in the diet to help prevent many chronic diseases, like cancer and heart disease. The antioxidants and fiber in many fruits and vegetables are essential for ensuring good health. But if food safety truly started with farm-based controls, consumers could enjoy the benefits of fresh produce without bearing the risk of becoming ill.

EGGS

Although *Salmonella* has long been associated with poultry products, including eggs, the hazards from eggs have actually increased in our lifetime. The hard shell around eggs should provide protection from bacterial contamination, and for years it did. So long as the eggs were clean and uncracked, consumers could feel confident that the yolk and the egg white inside the shell were sterile. But eggs provide a good illustration of the nature and challenge posed by living bacteria that can readily adapt to their environment.

HIDDEN EGGS

Eggs contaminated with *Salmonella* bacteria have caused hundreds of outbreaks of foodborne illness. Often, hidden egg ingredients are the culprits in outbreaks linked to other types of foods. Here are some examples of egg-containing foods that have caused outbreaks over the last ten years.

Ice cream

Hollandaise and béarnaise sauces

Crab dishes

Stuffing

Lasagna

Pie

Tiramisu

Source: Smith DeWaal et al., *Outbreak Alert!*, pp. 27–31.

Sometime in the 1970s or 1980s, a bacterium called *Salmonella* Enteritidis (SE) migrated into the ovaries of chickens.[45] From there, it contaminated eggs internally. Today, the government estimates that 1 egg in 20,000 holds the hazardous bacterium, which translates into about 2.3 million eggs annually. The problem is, there is no way for a consumer to tell which eggs are contaminated.[46]

While the egg industry says the hazard in eggs is insignificant,[47] the simple fact is that even one contaminated egg can trigger an outbreak. And once the bacterium gets into a restaurant or home kitchen that is insanitary, an outbreak can last for several weeks. For example, in June 1999, a number of people in Virginia became ill from *Salmonella*. After interviewing the food-poisoning victims, most of whom were elementary-aged children and teenagers, investigators determined that most of them had eaten at the International House of Pancakes in Richmond. In all, almost 180 people became ill from *Salmonella* over the course of a one-month period after eating in the restaurant. Local health officials closed the restaurant while they conducted food-handler training and an extensive cleanup of the restaurant.

The outbreak investigation disclosed many food-handling problems that allowed *Salmonella* to live in the restaurant environment for several weeks. Eggs were mixed together in large bowls or vats (a practice called pooling) and then kept overnight. The pooled eggs were then used to make omelettes or French toast.

The investigators concluded:

> Practices such as pooling raw eggs and allowing the pooled product to sit at room temperature, as was observed with the containers of raw pooled eggs, omelette mix and french toast batter, contributed to the outbreak. Also, it was unclear how frequently these containers were emptied and thoroughly cleaned; thus, after initial introduction of the organism into the restaurant, it could have persisted in the environment for a long time.[48]

Eggs are one of the most common foods to be linked to a food-poisoning outbreak. In fact, over 660,000 people are sickened and more than 300 are killed each year by SE-contaminated eggs. From 1990 to 2001, eggs and multi-ingredient egg dishes contaminated with SE were linked to over 200 outbreaks.

Although it started as a regional issue, the hazard posed by internally contaminated eggs has spread from coast to coast because of an ineffective system of regulating eggs. Today three different government agencies play a role in egg safety, and for years they either competed for jurisdiction or ignored the problem. That allowed the prevalence of *Salmonella* Enteritidis to increase in the flocks, thus increasing the risk to consumers of buying and eating infected eggs. Other countries have been much more aggressive in trying to eliminate this hazard by buying infected flocks from the producers and then destroying them.[49]

Because producers and the government failed to control this food-safety hazard, now consumers must. For example, when eggs used to be safer, it was okay for parents to let their children eat raw cookie dough. Today, that is no longer true.

SE illnesses can be fatal to vulnerable consumers such as the elderly, children, and those with suppressed immune systems. Unless SE-infected eggs are thoroughly cooked or pasteurized, the pathogens are not destroyed. Therefore, consumers should use pasteurized eggs when preparing foods that traditionally use raw eggs, such as Caesar salad dressing, tiramisu, meringue pies, mousses, and homemade ice cream. Pasteurized eggs also should be used in preparing dishes such as lasagna, baked ziti, puddings, or French toast, unless the eggs will be heated to a temperature of 145 degrees Fahrenheit.

If you use unpasteurized eggs, it is important to handle them safely. Keep eggs refrigerated at 40 degrees or less. Discard any cracked eggs. Use the eggs within a week of the sell-by date on the package, or, if there is no sell-by date, use the eggs within three weeks of purchase. Also, eggs that are fried or served sunny-side up should be cooked until the yolks are firm.

DAIRY

Dairy products were once a fairly common source of food-poisoning outbreaks. In fact, in 1938, milk outbreaks represented 25 percent of all food and water outbreaks. But with the advent of nearly universal pasteurization of milk, that number had fallen to 1 percent by 1993, which represents a tremendous public health improvement.[50]

Pasteurization is quite simple, requiring only that milk be heat-treated before it is sold.[51] Pasteurized milk is then used to produce all types of dairy products, such as bottled milk, cheeses, and yogurt.

In 1994, the single largest food-poisoning outbreak ever recorded in the United States occurred from a surprising product: ice cream. The ice cream was taken from one plant, where it was premixed, to the Schwan's Sales plant in Marshall, Minnesota, where it was frozen. Investigators believe the ice cream became contaminated in the tanker trucks that carried the premix. The trucks had previously carried liquid raw eggs, a common source of *Salmonella* Enteritidis. Although trucks that carry food are required to be washed between loads, that requirement generally goes unenforced. An investigation by the FDA showed that there were also cracks on the inside of the truck that couldn't be reached with standard washing. Whatever the cause, when the ice cream premix arrived at the Marshall plant, it was contaminated. There, it was frozen without being pasteurized a second time. The ice cream was sold door-to-door around the country and sickened an estimated 220,000 people in 41 states.[52]

Milk is regulated by the states under agreements with the federal

FIGURE 4
DAIRY OUTBREAKS, 1990–2001

Total number of reported outbreaks linked to dairy: 65

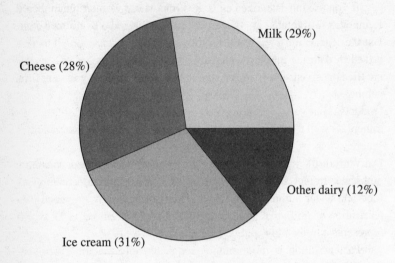

Milk (29%)

Cheese (28%)

Other dairy (12%)

Ice cream (31%)

Source: Smith DeWaal et al., *Outbreak Alert!*, p. 9.

government. Although popular in some areas, unpasteurized (or raw) milk is not sold over state lines.[53] While raw milk is still available in a few areas today, it is much too risky to drink. At least three potentially deadly hazards—*Listeria monocytogenes, Salmonella,* and *E. coli* O157:H7—can contaminate raw milk.

Some cheeses are made from unpasteurized milk, and cheese connoisseurs swear that they are stronger and more flavorful. Unfortunately, they have also been linked to illnesses and miscarriages from *Listeria* and at least one outbreak from *Salmonella*.[54]

In 1985, the FDA banned the sale of soft cheeses made from unpasteurized milk following a major outbreak linked to a Mexican-style soft cheese. That outbreak was one of the most deadly in our nation's history. *Listeria*-laden cheese caused 142 people to become ill, resulting in 48 deaths, mostly in the Hispanic community in southern California.[55]

That outbreak helped establish the link between *Listeria* and miscarriage. Researchers at the Los Angeles County USC Medical Center, the largest birthing center for Hispanic women in the United States, were studying factors causing spontaneous abortion and stillbirth. When the rates suddenly increased during the course of the study, researchers began questioning women to find out why. Many women remembered eating a specific brand of cheese that laboratory tests confirmed contained *Listeria.* This outbreak was the first time that foodborne bacteria had been linked to miscarriage.[56]

Raw (unpasteurized) milk and raw-milk cheeses have caused a number of outbreaks since 1990, so it is good practice to avoid those products. That is especially important for the youngest and oldest consumers, as well as pregnant women. Cheese made from pasteurized milk generally lists pasteurized milk among its ingredients.

While soft cheeses, like Brie or Camembert, made from unpasteurized milk have been banned for years, they are still found in many supermarkets. Hard cheeses such as cheddar, Colby, and Swiss can still be made from unpasteurized milk because those cheeses are aged for 60 days, which is widely believed to eliminate the hazard.[57] However, Canada recently had an outbreak linked to cheddar cheese, where *Salmonella* managed to survive the aging process. The FDA is currently doing research to determine whether hard cheeses made from unpasteurized milk pose a hazard to consumers. It is likely that research will identify a new, simple processing step that will ensure that these cheeses are safe, even when made with unpasteurized milk.

WILD CUISINE: SEAFOOD

With over 300 varieties of seafood for sale harvested from waters all over the world, seafood offers both unique nutritional benefits and a smorgasbord of hazards. Seafood is one of the only foods we consume regularly that is caught in the wild, although increasingly fish are being farmed as well. Seafood can contain an assortment of bacteria and parasites, hazards similar to those that plague meat and poultry products. In addition, seafood harbors some unique hazards from natural toxins and chemical contaminants.[58]

Despite these hazards, seafood processors are subject to much less

SHAPING A BETTER FOOD-SAFETY SYSTEM

When Carol Tucker Foreman discovered that the Bush administration was going to stop testing school lunch meat for *Salmonella,* her first call was to the *New York Times* and her second was to the *Washington Post.* Both papers ran front-page stories the next morning and Secretary of Agriculture Ann Veneman reversed the administration's course by 11 A.M., claiming that she was unaware of the policy change. Most advocates don't see the results of their work for years, but after nearly 30 years seeking food-safety improvements, Foreman doesn't like to wait. Though she has never lost her soft Arkansas drawl, Carol Tucker Foreman's message is heard loud and clear.

Foreman came to Washington from Arkansas and eventually became the executive director of the nonprofit Consumer Federation of America. Then in 1977, President Jimmy Carter appointed her assistant secretary of agriculture for food and consumer services. She had responsibility for a wide range of programs, including food stamps, school lunch programs, and the meat, poultry, and egg inspection programs. She also oversaw development of the first *Dietary Guidelines for Americans,* the nation's first basic nutrition policy.

Foreman's tenure at the USDA ended with the election of Ronald Reagan. "Shortly before the election, candidate Reagan promised the Texas Cattlefeeders Association that he would remove the consumer influence from USDA. He kept his promise," recalls Foreman. "He named a hog producer as secretary, and brought in a vice president of the National

oversight than their counterparts in the meat and poultry industry. Rather than daily or continuous inspection by the USDA, seafood processors are inspected once every one to two years by the FDA. That infrequent oversight has proven ineffective at improving conditions in the seafood-processing industry. For example, nearly three years after federal regulations required seafood processors to put new HACCP-based food-safety control systems in place, fewer than one-quarter of the processors had fully complied. Without far more government oversight and inspection, unsafe seafood will continue to harm consumers.

Seafood outbreaks are among the most common reported to the CDC. The Center for Science in the Public Interest's outbreak listings (compiled largely from CDC data) show the hazards most likely to cause

Cattlemen's Association to oversee meat and poultry inspection. Their views on food safety were just about what you'd expect."

Foreman refused to leave food-safety issues in the hands of the new administration and industry. In 1986, she launched a major campaign to revamp the archaic meat and poultry inspection system. She enlisted leading consumer, public health, and labor organizations to join her in forming the Safe Food Coalition. After 10 years of effort, the coalition succeeded in persuading the USDA to revamp its old "poke and sniff" inspection system, setting limits on disease-causing bacteria in meat and poultry products.

Foreman's leadership and wisdom over nearly 30 years have been instrumental in shaping the food-safety system of the future. In 1999, Foreman returned to the Consumer Federation of America as Distinguished Fellow and director of the Food Policy Institute. She remains ever watchful to ensure that government officials not forget that food safety is a critical consumer issue.

"It is time for the leadership at USDA to understand that a public-health-based inspection system for meat and poultry is both good economics and good politics," Carol Tucker Foreman says. "And American voters won't tolerate USDA putting the needs of cattlemen and giant companies before the public's health. The 76 million illnesses and 5,000 food-poisoning deaths each year provide persuasive arguments for clean products and a responsive system."

---

seafood-related outbreaks: scombroid and ciguatera (natural toxins that cause outbreaks from finfish), Norwalk virus, and *Vibrio* spp. and other bacteria frequently linked to shellfish.[59] Although smoked fish carry the deadly *Listeria* bacterium, there are few documented outbreaks linked to smoked fish. *Listeria* poses a special risk for pregnant women, immune-compromised individuals, and elderly consumers, but poses no risk to most healthy consumers.

Scombroid poisoning, one of the most common hazards associated with finfish, results from high levels of histamines that develop in fish that are not kept cold. In one particularly notable outbreak in 1997, 26 employees of the World Bank became violently ill from scombroid poisoning after eating blue marlin in the employees' cafeteria. The following

FIGURE 5
SEAFOOD HAZARDS, 1990–2001

Total number of reported outbreaks linked to seafood: 340

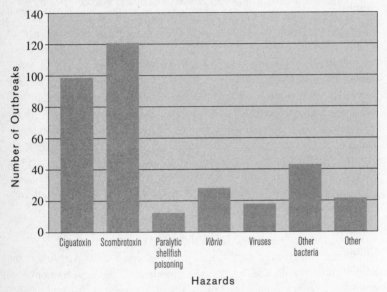

Source: Smith DeWaal el al., *Outbreak Alert!*, p. 17–21.

day, the *Washington Post* carried pictures of people on ambulance gur-
neys being taken out of the World Bank and rushed to the hospital. While
some might assume this outbreak was a case of international terrorism, it
was just another example of why the public needs tighter controls on
seafood.[60]

One of the best-known hazards in our food supply is from raw oysters. The old saying "Never eat oysters in a month without an 'r' in it"
turned out to have some scientific validity, although it didn't go far
enough. Gulf Coast waters provide a perfect environment for a host of
bacteria in the *Vibrio* family. Those bacteria multiply in the warm waters
of the Gulf, especially during the non-"r" summer months. One member
of this family, *Vibrio vulnificus,* is particularly deadly, killing about 15
to 20 people every year.[61] Unfortunately, the risk extends well into the
fall months.

Another strain of *Vibrio,* called *parahaemolyticus,* sickened over 400 people in 13 states in the summer of 1998. The culprits—contaminated oysters—were harvested from Galveston Bay, Texas. The Texas Health Department closed down the oyster beds in the area from June to November to stop the outbreak. It is likely that a ship had dumped its ballast waters in Galveston Bay, contaminating the harvesting beds with raw sewage that contained the bacteria.[62]

Other hazards from raw shellfish can easily show up in the winter months. For example, in January 1997, over 400 people in five states were sickened by oysters contaminated with the Norwalk virus. Following that outbreak, the CDC issued a report saying that the shellfish harvesters themselves may have contaminated the shellfish beds by throwing raw sewage overboard. Such lapses in sanitation clearly pose a significant public health risk and also point to lax government oversight of the shellfish industry.[63]

The regulation of shellfish is even weaker than that of finfish. The federal government has abdicated its responsibility for ensuring the safety of shellfish products to a body called the Interstate Shellfish Sanitation Conference. That group is made up of state regulators and shellfish producers primarily from shellfish-producing states.[64] They negotiate on state harvesting restrictions and other policies to ensure safe shellfish products. Unfortunately, through this conference, both state and federal officials regularly negotiate away public health standards in order to reach agreement with the industry. The conference has failed to develop policies that would remove the deadliest oysters from the marketplace and has stood in the way of other important changes that would improve the safety of shellfish products intended for raw consumption.

Given the current state of the regulation of shellfish, the best advice is to avoid raw oysters and clams from Gulf Coast waters unless they have been specially treated to remove harmful bacteria. Some approved treatments include a mild heat-pasteurization process and high pressure.[65]

For finfish, the advice is a little more complicated. Natural toxins in fish include both scombroid and ciguatera. Unlike bacteria, those toxins are heat-stable, which means they can't be cooked out of the fish. Ciguatera poisoning has many of the common symptoms of food poisoning, but it can also cause neurological symptoms. The classic symptom of ciguatera poisoning is a reversal of hot and cold on the tongue.[66] To cut your risk of ciguatera poisoning, avoid locally caught grouper, amber-jack, and red snapper when visiting tropical areas. That is especially a problem in Florida, the Caribbean, and Hawaii. Avoid barracuda every-where.

Scombroid poisoning is a potential problem for many types of fish, including fresh tuna, mackerel, mahimahi, sardines, and bluefish. Some people have reported that fish containing high levels of scombroid toxin taste peppery, but with many preparation methods that flavor would be unnoticeable. Symptoms include rash, headache, and itching (see Figure 1). The key to avoiding scombroid poisoning is to ensure that the fish is kept sufficiently cold from the time it leaves the water until the time it is cooked. Allowing fish to become warm for even a brief period can en-courage the development of histamines. Assuring the safety of fish today rests largely with the fish purveyor, due to the lax regulatory structure.[67] Check with your seafood supplier about the handling of fish before you buy it. Avoid buying seafood that is not well iced.

PRECAUTIONS TO TAKE WHEN EATING OUT

- Avoid raw oysters and clams from the Gulf Coast unless they have been treated to eliminate harmful bacteria.

- To cut your risk of ciguatera poisoning, avoid locally caught grouper, amberjack, and red snapper in tropical areas such as the Caribbean, Florida, and Hawaii. Avoid barracuda everywhere.

- Ask restaurants not to add raw sprouts to your sandwich or salad.

- Don't order your meat cooked rare or medium rare, and send it back if it is not cooked to order. Eat only medium-well or well-done meat.

- Don't order sunny-side-up or runny eggs. Eat eggs only if they are thoroughly cooked.

- If food is lukewarm when it reaches your table, send it back. Hot foods should be kept hot, and cold foods should be kept cold.

- The same holds true for buffets. Foods must be kept hotter or colder than the "danger zone" (40–140°F) in order to prevent bacterial growth.

- Use your best judgment: Don't eat at restaurants that aren't clean, and report insanitary conditions to the local health department.

STRONGER STANDARDS AND BETTER REGULATION

Many people play a role in keeping the food supply safe. Farmers and food processors can prevent hazards from entering food by improving controls both on the farm and in their factories. Restaurant and home chefs help eliminate hazards that enter the kitchen on raw food products. The government needs to develop and enforce strong standards to encourage the food industry to adopt the best practices to avoid food contamination.

Today, one food-safety agency regulates meat and poultry products, while another regulates all other foods including seafood, shell eggs, and dairy products. This patchwork of food-safety regulations creates many gaps in food-safety protections. For example:

- The use of animal manure on food crops has been linked to numerous food and waterborne outbreaks, but is subject to almost no oversight by the federal government.

- Issues like egg safety can remain unaddressed for over a decade because shared jurisdiction prevents the development of needed regulations.

- Inspection resources are being duplicated in some areas and are completely absent in other areas.

- The quality of new programs to improve food safety, like the HACCP programs for meat, poultry, and seafood, vary widely, depending on whether they are administered by the FDA or the USDA.

- Imported products are treated entirely differently depending on whether the FDA or the USDA has jurisdiction over them.

In 1998, the National Academy of Sciences (NAS; the official scientific advisory body for the federal government) reviewed America's food-safety system and, in a report entitled *Ensuring Safe Food from Production to Consumption,* concluded that the "current fragmented regulatory structure is not well equipped to meet the current challenges."[68]

The public shouldn't have to wait for more preventable outbreaks and unnecessary deaths to illustrate the gaps in our federal programs.

New food-safety hazards, like *E. coli* O157:H7, increasing imports of food products, and the urgent need for more on-farm food-safety practices have amply demonstrated the weaknesses in the present system. Federal food-safety efforts should be unified under a single agency with broad oversight and strong enforcement authority.

IF YOU GET SICK

Most foodborne illnesses require no treatment other than fluids and rest. But drinking fluids may not be so easy when you are throwing up every 10 minutes.

"Try drinking small quantities frequently," says physician Glenn Morris of the University of Maryland. Even a sip or two every few minutes can keep you from getting dehydrated. "Fluids like Pedialyte are best, but other clear liquids like ginger ale or apple juice may also help. People get into trouble when they don't keep up with the fluid loss," adds Morris. "Even though you lose liquids when you throw up there's a net gain."

If you want something to reduce a fever, says Morris, take acetaminophen (Tylenol) rather then aspirin or ibuprofen (Advil), which could irritate your stomach. But call the doctor if you experience any of the following symptoms:

- **Bloody diarrhea or pus in the stool.** "They generally are signs of bacterial infection with organisms like *E. coli* O157:H7, *Campylobacter*, or *Shigella*," says Morris. "While you may not need antibiotics, it's a good idea to check with your doctor."

- **Fever that lasts more than 48 hours.** In adults it could signal an infection that's not getting better. Children are far more likely to develop nonthreatening fevers that last more than a day or two.

- **Faintness, rapid heart rate, or dizziness after sitting or standing up suddenly, or a significant drop in the frequency of urination.** This could mean life-threatening dehydration.

One final suggestion: Getting a stool culture is the only way to find out what caused your illness and help public health officials identify an outbreak. If you suspect that you have food poisoning or your doctor confirms it, call your local health department. You can search for health departments on the web at www.nascio.org/stateSearch/displayCategory.cfm?Category=health.

ANOTHER REASON FOR STRONGER GOVERNMENT OVERSIGHT: BIOTERRORISM AND THE FOOD SUPPLY

The September 11, 2001, terrorist attack on the United States, followed by anthrax-laced letters sent to government and media offices, spurred widespread concern about the vulnerability of our food supply to acts of intentional contamination, as well as concern about the ability of our nation's food-safety system to minimize the risks. In the weeks that followed those events, Secretary of Health and Human Services Tommy Thompson told Congress that the safety of the food supply was one of his top concerns.

A CDC strategic-planning workgroup had previously concluded in 2000 that terrorists might try to contaminate our food supply using deadly pathogens such as *Clostridium botulinum* or *E. coli* O157:H7. A recent NAS report agreed, explaining that biological agents can be produced relatively quickly and inexpensively and without technical skill. In a 1984 bioterrorist event, harmful bacteria were used by a religious commune in Oregon to try to impact an election. Members of the commune contaminated 10 restaurant salad bars with *Salmonella* Typhimurium, sickening 751 people.[69]

Even more frightening is the possibility of terrorists' contaminating a common food source that is widely distributed. Most imported food is shipped into the United States with no inspection and then rapidly distributed around the country. If an imported food was used in a bioterrorist event, it might take weeks or even months for public health officials to recognize the food source and remove it from the stores. Also, it would be hard to prevent the airborne contamination of a large farm field or a water supply in the United States.

Bioterrorism is just the latest example of the problem with relying on old laws to regulate new hazards. The deficiencies in our federal food-safety system have left consumers—and the food industry itself—vulnerable. The FDA, for example, inspects only a small fraction of imported food shipments because it has just a few hundred inspectors responsible for ensuring the safety of 4 million shipments of imported foods. In addition, the FDA has about 1,000 food inspectors to check

57,000 food-processing plants. By contrast, the USDA has approximately 7,600 inspection personnel for about 6,500 meat, poultry, and processed-egg plants.

The responsibility for food safety is split among 12 federal agencies, from the Department of Agriculture to the Bureau of Alcohol, Tobacco, and Firearms. Balkanization and inflexible restrictions on applying resources result in many gaps and inconsistencies in government oversight. A stronger federal food-safety system is an essential component of a defense against terrorist attacks on the food supply and also would help to prevent foodborne illnesses due to unintentional product contamination.

Whether the problem is intentional food contamination by bioterrorists or unintentional contamination in a dirty food plant, our food-safety system is flawed. The challenges are so great, in fact, that they led Professor John Bailar, the chair of the NAS committee that wrote *Ensuring Safe Food from Production to Consumption,* to conclude: "Our country needs a single independent food safety agency. . . . When bioterrorism is added to the mix, the case for prompt and sweeping change becomes compelling."[70]

CHAPTER THREE

EATING FOR THE ENVIRONMENT

For many people, the quintessential environmental moment at the grocery store comes at the end when the bagger asks that age-old question: "Paper or plastic?" Well-intentioned shoppers have spent countless anxious moments trying to decide how to answer. Should they choose paper because it's a natural, renewable, easily recycled material? Or is plastic better because it's lighter and requires fewer raw materials to make?

Numerous lengthy studies have tried to prove that one of the two options is better than the other. But, in reality, this decision is one of the least significant environmental choices you make at the food store. In fact, neither alternative is significantly better than the other, and you can choose whichever you find most convenient.

Rather than worrying about the environment at the checkout counter, think about it instead when deciding which foods to put in the shopping cart. Although food choices have generally received little attention from environmental groups, food is one of the three largest consumer-related causes of environmental problems, along with cars and home energy use.

To protect natural habitats, preserve precious water supplies, slow global warming, and reduce sickness from contaminated water, we need to change the ways in which our society grows and consumes food. While many changes are needed at the government and farm level, consumers can also play an essential role in moving American society toward a safer, more environmentally sound food system.

This chapter examines how the current food system damages the environment and what can be done about it. It explains which foods to avoid—as well as which to eat—if you want a safer, healthier environment. It will evaluate various food choices solely in terms of their environmental impacts, but, as we will see later, there is considerable overlap between foods that are good for the environment and those that are good for your personal health.

WOULD YOU LIKE SOME POLLUTED WATER WITH THOSE FRIES TODAY?

The Consumer's Guide to Effective Environmental Choices,[1] published in 1999, was the first-ever comprehensive study of the environmental impacts of everything American consumers buy and do. It looked at how much air pollution, water pollution, and other environmental problems were caused by the purchase and use of such diverse products as paints, poultry, and plumbing fixtures. In fact, it divided consumer spending into 134 such different categories.

This book traced everything back from the end user—the consumer—through the manufacturing and distribution processes. In the case of cars, the most damaging of the 134 categories, the book considered the pollution caused by making steel, plastic, and rubber for new cars, as well as the energy required to ship those cars to dealers' showrooms, the paper used by car companies for sales brochures, and the pollution cars produce when they burn gasoline. In the case of pasta, the book factored in everything from the water, the fertilizers, and the pesticides used to grow the wheat, to the electricity used at the food-processing facility where the wheat is manufactured into spaghetti, to the diesel fuel used by the trucks that ship the boxes of pasta to the food store.

When compared with nine other big consumer-spending categories, such as health care and housing, food scored stunningly high. It was responsible for more water pollution, water use, and land-related impacts than any of the other categories. To illustrate some of the serious ways in which food production and consumption can harm the environment, let's imagine a typical day's food.

For breakfast, you might choose that old standby—corn flakes—and unwittingly contribute to the so-called "dead zone" in the Gulf of Mexico. The corn in the cereal likely comes from Iowa or elsewhere in the Midwest corn belt. Over the past decades, farmers have dramatically increased the amount of corn they get off an acre of land—from 29 bushels in 1940 to 137 bushels today.[2] But one of the ways they've accomplished that is by spreading large quantities of chemical nitrogen fertilizers on their fields. Some of that fertilizer washes off the fields and into nearby streams, while some evaporates into the atmosphere. In both cases, a portion of it finds its way down the Mississippi River basin and into the Gulf of Mexico, where it joins nitrogen from sewage, power plants, and other sources.

Just as the nitrogen boosts plant growth on croplands, it increases algae growth in the water, making it murkier. When the algae die and decompose, oxygen levels in the water fall, killing or driving off fish, shellfish, and other sea life, and creating a large area where little can live. During the 1990s, the Gulf of Mexico dead zone more than doubled in size to an area roughly as large as New Jersey. If current trends continue, this sort of environmental damage around the world will increase 2.5 times over the next 50 years.[3]

Your lunch causes yet more water pollution if you decide to eat a ham sandwich. Some of the waste from the pig ends up in the water supply. Each year, livestock generate 2 billion tons of wet manure. That's 10 times more than the amount of municipal solid waste and works out to 20 tons for every household in the country! Although human waste is subjected to multiple treatments before it is released into the environment, much of the manure ends up in the environment completely untreated, contributing to pollution and food-safety problems.

In recent years, not only the quantity of animal waste has been a problem, but so has its concentration on ever-larger livestock farms that operate on a scale radically different from a traditional family farm. As a report on these facilities points out, "Today's large livestock operations look more like animal factories than animal farms." A single hog facility can include tens of thousands of hogs in dozens of massive steel barns, while the biggest poultry farms have hundreds of thousands of chickens. With facilities that large, the smell can permeate the surroundings. In the case of Perryton, Texas, the odor of manure travels downwind for 15 miles. People have to keep their windows closed, and nearby neighbors claim the smell is so bad that it literally makes them sick.[4]

Disposing of the massive quantities of animal waste is an even bigger concern. When something goes wrong, the consequences can be disastrous. The waste is frequently stored in open-air pits called lagoons, many larger than an acre. In April 1999, a hole opened in one such lagoon at a giant hog farm in Duplin County, North Carolina. Through the hole, 1.5 million gallons of manure and urine flowed into a wetlands next to a tributary of the Northeast Cape Fear River, killing fish and other wildlife. That year, there were more than 100 other significant animal waste spills, although on a smaller scale than Duplin County's. But that year was by no means unique. The previous year, a spill dumped 100,000 gallons of hog waste into Minnesota's Beaver Creek, killing nearly 700,000 fish.[5]

But let's get back to the hypothetical day's food. For dinner, you won't have to worry about the impacts of animal agriculture, since you decide to grill up some mako shark. Not only does the charcoal grill contribute to air pollution, but eating shark helps wipe out the world's shark population. Although movies like *Jaws* suggest that sharks are a threat to humans, in reality it's almost always the other way around. According to the National Audubon Society, "Each year, sharks kill fewer than a dozen people worldwide. But people kill more than 100 million sharks."[6] The surviving population is declining rapidly and it will be difficult for their numbers to rebound, since sharks mature slowly and have few offspring.

RUNNING THE NUMBERS

To understand how consumers can most effectively reduce the environmental damage associated with food, it is important to move beyond dramatic examples to some general data. Figure 6, based on the data in *The Consumer's Guide to Effective Environmental Choices,* summarizes food's share of Americans' total environmental impacts.[7] Clearly, the greatest food-related impacts come from the use of critical resources— water and land. When Americans think about ways to conserve water, they generally focus on using less on their lawns and in household activities, such as taking showers and doing the laundry. Although such water-saving measures are useful, nearly three-quarters of all the water consumers use goes to providing them with food—primarily for irrigating farmers' fields.

The "land use" category is important because if society is to preserve the rich biodiversity of nature, we need large amounts of land where wild plants and animals can thrive. To come up with the land-use impact per-

FIGURE 6
FOOD: ITS SHARE OF CONSUMERS' TOTAL IMPACTS

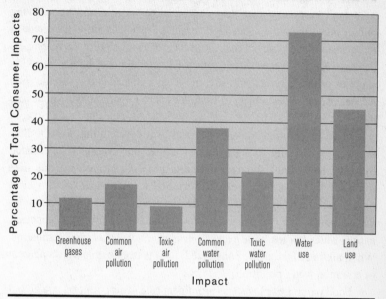

centage in the graph, *The Consumer's Guide* ranked various land uses differently, acre for acre, with farmers' fields by no means being the most harmful to nature. A much wider range of wild plants and animals can coexist with farms than with city office blocks or parking lots, for example. Nevertheless, because so much more land is used for farming, the total impact on wildlife is high—45 percent of consumers' total land-related impact, according to this approach.

Water pollution is the third most important way that Americans' food choices harm the environment. One can draw a distinction between two different types of water pollution—toxic and common. Food production contributes significantly to both of them. Toxic water pollution is most often associated with heavy industry—discharges from petro-chemical factories and heavy metals, such as mercury, lead, and cadmium. These chemicals can contaminate drinking water, kill plant life, and contaminate fish. But food is responsible for about 22 percent of the

toxic water pollution, primarily because of the widespread use of pesticides on farmers' fields. Pesticides—whether they are herbicides, insecticides, or fungicides—are expressly designed to kill living organisms,
so it isn't surprising that they can endanger people and harm living
things other than their intended targets. Pesticides pose the greatest
threat to farmworkers, but their impact extends much further. When pesticides wash off farmers' fields, they can contaminate human drinking
supplies or lakes, rivers, and streams. They can also end up on the food
we eat. (Because the subject of pesticides is so important, we will devote
most of chapter 4 to it.)

In addition to highly toxic chemicals, various common water pollutants can be harmful to people and wildlife. For example, soil eroded
from cropland, rangeland, recently logged forests, and construction sites
frequently winds up in lakes, streams, and coastal waters. That runoff
makes the water cloudy, affecting the penetration of sunlight and chok-
ing off plants. Fertilizers and livestock waste wash off farms, contaminating water bodies with excess nitrogen, phosphates, and sediments.
When all these factors are considered, food is responsible for 38 percent
of common water pollution.

Food purchases play a less prominent role in air pollution and global
warming, though they are certainly still not insignificant. As with water
pollution, we can distinguish between two types of air pollution—
common and toxic. Food is responsible for 17 percent of the former and
9 percent of the latter. Some comes from burning gasoline and other
fuels in tractors and other farm equipment, and for heating and lighting
barns and other farm buildings. But other significant sources of this air
pollution can be traced to manufacturing fertilizers and pesticides, to
processing food, and to shipping food to stores and restaurants.

Food is responsible for 12 percent of consumers' total global warming impact. Many of the same things that cause air pollution also cause
global warming. However, the shipping of foods to market plays a greater
role—about one-quarter of the total food impact on global warming.

Given the large role that food plays in our lives, its high environmental impacts are understandable. In terms of sheer weight, much of
what Americans use on a daily basis is food. Although people worry
about whether to choose paper or plastic bags at the grocery store, those

items don't require very much in the way of materials. If you were to choose plastic bags and then save them all for an entire year, you might have 8 pounds' worth by the end. In comparison, an average American annually uses 582 pounds of dairy products, 65 pounds of beef, 51 pounds of chicken, and 281 pounds of fruit, plus large quantities of vegetables, grains, and other products (see Appendix A). It isn't surprising that growing, processing, and shipping all this food would have a wide range of impacts on the environment.

While food production will always require considerable land and more water than any other human activity, the environmental damage could be dramatically reduced. We could have a food system that ensures that pesticides don't get into drinking water or poison farmworkers and that uses water much more efficiently, preserves valuable topsoil, keeps animal waste out of rivers, and prevents the extinction of fish species.

THE CONSUMER'S ROLE

For those improvements to happen, the government will need to give much more attention to reducing the environmental impacts of agriculture, while farmers will need to change some of their common practices. But consumers shouldn't passively wait for industry and government to deliver a better food system. Through our personal food choices, we can directly reduce pollution and also send clear signals to grocery stores, restaurants, farmers, food processors, and the government, letting them know that we want a food system that is better for both the environment and our health.

For one thing, not all food has the same impacts. Some of the foods we eat cause much more harm to the environment than others. If we reduced our consumption of those foods that cause the most environmental damage, and ate more of the environment-friendly foods, it would have huge environmental benefits. The most important actions individuals could take would be to eat less meat, choose organic foods, and promote sustainable fishing.

THREE KEY STEPS FOR THE ENVIRONMENT
Eat less meat.
Choose organic foods.
Promote sustainable fishing.

EAT LESS MEAT

For the average American, the most important and most useful step is to eat less meat. You don't need to become a vegetarian, but reducing meat consumption—or even switching from beef and pork to poultry—would have important environmental paybacks. Thankfully, this advice will not only help the environment; it will also improve your health.

To see why reducing meat consumption is so desirable, let's compare eating hamburger or chicken with eating rice. Even without doing any analysis, we would expect the rice to be somewhat better, because of the simple fact that it's more efficient for people to consume grains directly than livestock that have been raised on grains. Most of the grain the animals eat does not get converted to edible meat.

But when we quantify the differences, some of the numbers turn out to be much more dramatic than one might expect. Figure 7 compares the environmental impacts of a pound of rice with a pound of hamburger with a pound of chicken.[8] We have assigned the various impacts of the rice a score of "1." The bars on the figure for the hamburger and the chicken show how much worse the impacts of those meats are. In most categories, the impacts of eating hamburger are many times worse than the impacts of eating rice. The land-use impacts are more than 16 times worse, not only because of the inefficiency of feeding grain to cattle, but because of cattle grazing. Because cattle waste sometimes contaminates water supplies, the common water-pollution impacts are more than 17 times worse. Chemicals applied to feed grains cause more than a fivefold increase in toxic water pollution. Greater energy use and methane emissions from cattle's belching mean that the hamburger generates more than 5 times the greenhouse gases that contribute to global warming. And even in the water-use and air-pollution categories, where the differences aren't as great, beef is more than 3 times worse

FIGURE 7
RICE VERSUS CHICKEN VERSUS HAMBURGER

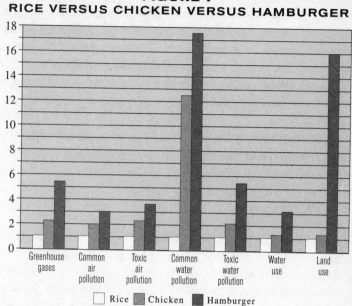

☐ Rice ▨ Chicken ■ Hamburger

than rice. Of course, beef provides considerably more protein than rice, but there's no getting around the fact that it's many times worse for the environment.

Surprisingly, chicken is closer to rice than to beef in most categories. In fact, the numbers for water use and land use are fairly comparable for rice and chicken. But because of the chicken's waste, common water pollution is more than 12 times worse than for rice.

When pasta rather than rice is compared with chicken and hamburger, the results are similar, although pasta does even better than rice in the water-use category because growing rice is relatively water intensive. Pasta requires slightly less than half the water of rice and chicken, and only one-seventh as much water as hamburger. In most of the other categories, rice and pasta are relatively comparable, so eating either one is clearly better for the environment than eating meat.[9]

What all these numbers mean is that it does indeed make a difference what we eat. Clearly, reducing meat consumption would significantly improve environmental quality. But this doesn't mean that you need to become a vegetarian for environmental reasons. To understand why, let's assume you currently have an average American diet, including more than one pound (boneless) of chicken and more than two pounds (boneless) of beef and pork per week. If you were to cut chicken consumption to three-quarters of a pound, and beef and pork consumption to a quarter pound, you would achieve about 80 percent of the environmental improvement of eliminating meat entirely from your diet. Getting rid of that last pound of weekly meat consumption would have only a fairly small environmental benefit. You may reasonably decide that you enjoy meat enough that you want to keep some of it in your diet, or you may decide to go all the way.

Eat Better Meat

If you decide to keep eating modest quantities of beef, chicken, and other meat, you can further reduce the environmental impacts by carefully choosing what you buy. Some meat is raised in ways that cause much less harm to the environment than others. Once new federal regulations on organic foods go into effect in October 2002, you can look for certified, organically raised meat. Meat with the USDA organic label will come from animals that haven't been routinely fed antibiotics and growth hormones, and whose feed wasn't grown with synthetic pesticides or fertilizers. In addition, the animals will not have been confined to crowded, indoor factory farms or feedlots that leave the animals susceptible to disease. Organically raised animals are required by the guidelines to have access to the outdoors.

Because the standards for organic meat are quite stringent, there may initially be a limited supply. Therefore, look for other meat that you can tell was produced in an environmentally sound way. For example, look for meat labeled "antibiotic-free," not only because rampant antibiotic use in animal feed is a serious problem in its own right, as we saw in chapter 2, but because antibiotic-free meat is often produced on farms with less crowding, so that animal diseases can't spread easily. Free-range chickens are often another good choice, although the actual environmental benefits vary greatly since producers can meet this standard by giving their chickens as little as five minutes of open-air access daily.

Just don't be seduced by vague, meaningless terms like "natural" or by producers who claim they are environmentally sound, but give you no evidence to prove it. Also, ignore a label of "no hormones administered" on pork and poultry, since the U.S. Department of Agriculture prohibits hormones from being given to any pork or poultry. If you can't decide whether a claim or a label is meaningful or not, you can look it up on www.eco-labels.org, a helpful website developed by Consumers Union, the organization that publishes *Consumer Reports*. They'll tell you who or what is behind the label and whether the claim means anything or not.

Make Your Voice Heard

Purchasing less meat is only part of the solution. You can also let your elected representatives and other policymakers know that you want state and federal governments to take steps to reduce environmental damage from meat production. Here are two key things the government could do.

1. Reduce pollution from animal waste

Farmers have traditionally viewed manure as a valuable resource for fertilizing their fields. Indeed, organic farmers rely heavily on manure, because they seek to avoid chemical fertilizers. But for many of the large livestock facilities, animal waste is a serious problem rather than a valuable resource. The facilities produce so much that it is costly and difficult to dispose of it all safely.

Take our prior example, Duplin County, North Carolina, where the 1.5-million-gallon waste spill occurred. In this one county, with just 42,000 people, there are 2.2 million hogs, and several million tons of waste is produced annually. The manure is placed into open-pit lagoons that are designed to allow it to break down into simpler compounds for use as fertilizer. Unfortunately, some of the waste regularly leaks out of the lagoons, many of which are unlined, into the groundwater, which then feeds into drinking wells. A study of groundwater in North Carolina found that 38 percent of the sites near unlined hog lagoons had been sufficiently polluted to contaminate nearby wells with *E. coli* and other bacteria that indicate fecal contamination. A different study by the state showed that lining the lagoons wouldn't solve this problem, since a quarter of lined facilities leaked and contaminated groundwater.[10]

Even if there were no leaks from the lagoons, the next step in the process would still be problematic. After the hog waste breaks down into a liquid, it is sprayed as fertilizer onto fields. The lagoon system doesn't eliminate pathogens, and the fertilizer it produces continues to have pathogen levels 100 to 10,000 times higher than human waste that is applied to land after processing at a municipal waste-treatment facility.[11] Moreover, the quantities of hog waste are so large that some waste inevitably runs off into nearby lakes, rivers, and streams, especially during spring and summer rains. When there's flooding, as during Hurricane Floyd in 1999, waste filled with microbial pathogens flows from the fields and lagoons into nearby rivers.

The manure contaminates the air as well as the water due to the emission of large quantities of ammonia. The amount of ammonia in rain doubled between the mid-1980s and mid-1990s in those parts of North Carolina where large hog factories were built.[12]

To deal with those problems, not just in North Carolina, but also in the many other states with large-scale livestock operations, the open lagoons should be phased out and replaced by newer technologies. States like North Carolina have taken some promising first steps but need to do more. A recent economic analysis by the nonprofit group Environmental Defense shows that much safer waste-management technologies could be put in place for three cents or less per pound of pork, and society would save significant water cleanup and healthcare costs.[13]

In general, the government needs to establish strong environmental and health standards for large livestock facilities. Those farms should be kept out of floodplains, away from wetlands, and apart from other sensitive lands. They should be required to monitor nearby water quality to make sure that they are not polluting. In addition, farmers should be encouraged to change the composition of livestock feed in ways that would reduce odor and emissions of ammonia.[14]

Even the largest facilities could be much safer and healthier. For example, the Perdue chicken company has built a waste-processing plant in Delaware that will annually convert 94,000 tons of chicken manure to pasteurized pellets that can be shipped to Midwest farms for use as fertilizer. That means that less chicken waste will end up in Chesapeake Bay.

2. Eliminate overgrazing on federal lands

Cattle graze on tens of millions of acres across the American West, before they usually spend the last few months of their lives in factory-farm-like feedlots. Although grazing eliminates the environmental impacts of growing grain for feed, it can have other environmental costs. Cattle trample plants and compact the soil, sometimes making it difficult for various types of plants to grow. As a result, in some places nonindigenous invasive weeds replace native grasses and plants. Because devegetated, compacted land can't absorb as much water, runoff and soil erosion increase. Some native animals lose their food sources. In the worst situations, the land takes decades or centuries to recover, even after grazing ends.

Cattle grazing doesn't have to be so destructive, however. Instead of allowing the cattle to roam over an entire ranch, permitting them to overgraze their favorite places, ranchers can divide a pasture into smaller sections, periodically moving the cattle to a new area when the previous one needs a rest. As one advocate of this sort of rotational grazing points out, this method also fertilizes the land by spreading the cattle's manure evenly over it: "This allows nutrients to be cycled more uniformly across the land, rather than being too concentrated in one area, while other areas receive little."[15]

As long as rotational grazing and other low-impact practices are used, there is no reason to eliminate all grazing. Well-managed, profitable cattle ranches should be encouraged to continue in parts of the West, since their demise would cause open land to be replaced by suburban houses and commercial development. Moreover, cattle can be raised on land that is unsuitable for other farming, thereby increasing the total food supply.

The federal government could eliminate practices that degrade public lands. Across the West, cattle graze on more than 2 million acres of federal land managed by the U.S. Forest Service and the Bureau of Land Management. In many places, the federal government subsidizes cattle ranching by leasing land at below-market rates (costing taxpayers about $100 million per year) and not insisting on grazing practices that maintain land quality. Although land degradation may be no worse on those public lands than on private ranches, the federal government has a responsibility to preserve its lands for future generations and to protect natural habitats. Yet according to the Bureau of Land Management's own statistics, half of the land it is responsible for is in poor or fair condition, much of it because of poor grazing practices in prior generations.[16] Strong pressure from ranching interests has discouraged the government from moving as fast or as far as it could to protect these lands. The government needs to keep cattle off the most vulnerable properties, require the best management practices, and prevent abuses. Because only a small fraction of the nation's meat production comes from cattle raised on federal lands, the nation's food supply would be little affected.

The Dairy Case

Milk, cheese, and other dairy items are products of animal agriculture, but are they as bad for the environment as meat? In general, they aren't, because they are produced more efficiently. Only 10 percent of the cattle in the United States are dairy cows, but their production of milk, by

---

SELLING FOOD WITH A MESSAGE

Gary Hirshberg went into the yogurt business to raise money for an education project, but then he realized that the business itself could be a vehicle for public education.

Hirshberg joined Stonyfield Farm as president in 1983, a few months after organic-agriculture pioneer Samuel Kayman started the farm to teach people about where their food came from. Hirshberg and Kayman were soon selling the yogurt they produced from their seven Jersey cows.

Gradually, Hirshberg built the nation's fourth-largest yogurt company, but he didn't forget his initial educational mission. With the company's products entering the homes of literally millions of people, Stonyfield Farm has been able to spread information about the environment, food safety, and nutrition.

Hirshberg's most creative and visible educational outreach effort turns the lids of the company's yogurt containers into message boards that encourage consumers to take action on environmental issues. As Hirshberg notes, "These little billboards allow us to fulfill our educational mission without taking away from what's in the cup." Through the lids, Stonyfield Farm has urged yogurt eaters to ask the federal government to prohibit antibiotics in organic foods and to push the president to address global warming. Consumers have also received tips on reducing their own use of toxic chemicals and energy.

weight, is 3.5 times greater than the production of beef and beef products. A dairy cow can annually produce many times its own weight in milk. Of course, most of that is water, but if we take that into consideration and compare the amount of protein produced, dairy production still converts feed grains and other inputs into usable food for humans much more efficiently than meat production does.

Nevertheless, some of the large dairy farms in California and elsewhere cause the same sorts of water pollution and animal-waste problems as the factory hog farms in North Carolina. And, on average, dairy production causes more environmental damage than fruits, vegetables, and grains. You can help the environment by changing to organic dairy products. Cows on organic farms eat feed grown without pesticides and do not receive antibiotics as routine supplements.

The company uses more than its lids to educate. It distributes a free guide to understanding what organic agriculture is and a monthly "moosletter" with health and nutrition information. It provides kids and teachers with environmental education activity kits and audiocassettes.

Because consumers are rightly skeptical of the motives of companies that claim to be concerned about environment quality, Hirshberg has had to be vigilant to ensure that Stonyfield Farm practices what it preaches. He reduced the environmental impacts of the company's manufacturing processes by increasing energy efficiency, choosing environmentally friendly building materials for the factory, and switching to a better type of plastic container. The company paid for reforestation to address global warming and produced a free guide showing other businesses how to reduce their greenhouse gas emissions. It also provides grants that promote sustainable farming practices and contributes 10 percent of its profits to environmental organizations.

These sorts of activities have been the foundation of the company's impressive growth, since they helped Stonyfield Farm forge an emotional bond with its customers and increased their loyalty. Although he recently sold the company to the large corporation that markets Dannon yogurt, Hirshberg hopes to maintain this bond. He advises other business leaders that "doing good in and with your company can be the most empowering and financially successful strategy you can implement."

BUY ORGANIC FRUITS, VEGETABLES, AND GRAINS

Nutritionists encourage us to make fruits, vegetables, and grains the core of our diet. Although those foods cause less environmental damage than meat, that doesn't mean their impacts are insignificant. Pesticides and chemical fertilizers used on crops pollute the nation's drinking water, as well as lakes, rivers, and bays. In addition, conventional farming practices deplete two essential, but limited, resources—topsoil and freshwater.

On many farms, environmentally damaging practices build on each other. Because water is often provided by the government at low subsidized rates, farmers have little incentive to conserve it. In California, so much water is taken from rivers, streams, and wetlands that some fish and wildlife can't survive. In the High Plains from Texas to Nebraska, farmers are drawing down water so fast from the underground Ogallala Aquifer that some places will have little left for future generations. When water is used profligately, much of it runs off the farm, transporting dangerous chemicals into rivers and streams. Studies by the California state government and the U.S. Department of Agriculture have shown that inefficient use of water by farmers unnecessarily increases the amounts of pesticides and toxic chemicals, such as selenium, in drinking water and rivers.[17]

To lessen these farm-based problems, make sure that at least some of the fruits, vegetables, and grains you buy are organically grown. Purchasing organic food not only directly reduces some environmental impacts, but also sends a powerful message to supermarkets, food processors, farmers, and the government—that the food supply should be safe for you and the environment.

Sales of organic products in the United States have been going up by about 20 percent a year. Nevertheless, only a small share of our food is grown organically. European Union agriculture has moved more decisively toward organics—it's currently around 2 percent of the total, or twice the U.S. total, and expected to be 10 to 30 percent by 2010—but the United States can catch up if consumers demand more organic products.

Organic agriculture is the best known of a variety of approaches farmers are taking to reduce agriculture's environmental impacts. Organic farmers abstain from using all synthetic pesticides and fertilizers.

They also reject irradiation, sewage sludge as fertilizer, and genetically engineered crops.

Other farmers who share the goal of reducing the environmental costs of agriculture may continue to use chemical inputs, but at reduced levels. They practice "integrated pest management," which means they don't routinely spray chemical pesticides, but instead try whenever possible to control pests through nonchemical means, such as using pest-eating insects like ladybugs. More important, they take steps to prevent pests from gaining a foothold in their fields in the first place. By planting different crops in successive years, they discourage insect pests that like only one crop. Farmers won't have as big a problem with European corn borers, for example, if they don't grow corn year after year. Crop rotation also has another benefit: planting legumes like soybeans builds nitrogen in the soil, reducing the need to apply chemical nitrogen fertilizers. This reduces water pollution and cuts down on air pollution and global warming associated with manufacturing fertilizer.[18]

Organic and other sustainable farmers give special attention to improving the quality of their soil. As several scientists noted in an article on sustainable agriculture in *Scientific American,* "To understand the rationale for sustainable agriculture, one must grasp the critical importance of soil. . . . [I]t is a complex, living, fragile medium that must be protected and nurtured to ensure its long-term productivity and stability." Because conventional agriculture may kill vital microorganisms in the soil and allows valuable topsoil to run off into nearby rivers and streams, farmers converting to sustainable practices often face a time-consuming and costly process of soil rebuilding. On farms in the prairie states, about half of the 10 inches of topsoil has been lost over the past century, so it's important to preserve this valuable resource.[19]

Although organic farmers are sometimes pictured as back-to-nature hippies trying to return to the traditional agricultural practices of the nineteenth century, organic agriculture is actually a highly sophisticated, scientifically based enterprise. It's not easy to control pests and increase productivity without relying on the chemical crutches of conventional agriculture. Successful organic farmers need to develop complex understandings of how various crops, pests, pest predators, beneficial animals, and microorganisms can interact with their particular soil and climate to produce the most food at the least cost and with the fewest problems.

Until recently, organic farmers received virtually no technical support from government agencies or agricultural colleges. An analysis of 4,500 research projects funded by the U.S. Department of Agriculture in 1995 found that only 34 focused explicitly on organic agriculture.[20] Fortunately, government and university researchers have recently begun providing more help.

With so little help, it's impressive how successful many organic farmers have been. Some have very large operations. Some long-established organic farmers, both large and small, are able to produce just as much food per acre as their conventional counterparts, and they have higher profit levels because they avoid the cost of chemical inputs and can charge a premium for their products.

That doesn't mean that organic farms will be able to produce the same yields and profits as conventional farms in all situations. The evidence up to now suggests that the success of organic methods will vary with the crop and the location. For example, at least two solid comparative studies—one in California and one in Washington—show that it would make economic as well as environmental sense to convert most apple production along the West Coast to organic methods. In the California test case, the organic trees produced more apples per tree, but they didn't grow quite as large. Because of more total fruit and higher prices for the organic apples, profits were higher. In Washington, not only were yields comparable, but the organic field had better soil quality and fewer environmental impacts.[21] Winegrowers like California's Fetzer's Vineyards have been similarly successful. For two decades, the Rodale Institute has compared test plots using organic and conventional methods, with impressive results. They found that especially when there is a drought or other "less-than-optimal growing conditions," organic methods can outproduce conventional ones.[22]

In contrast, some organic vegetable farmers in the East have experienced more problems. In Switzerland, in a rigorous 21-year trial conducted by the Research Institute of Organic Agriculture, organic fields experienced an average crop-yield reduction of 20 percent.[23] Although that is higher than other studies have shown, there will undoubtedly be some decline in total food produced, because organic farmers' crop rotations mean that fields are sometimes given over to less productive crops.

Opponents of organic agriculture seize on any negative food production data to argue that organic agriculture would be bad for the environment because it would require more land than conventional farming. Although organic agriculture currently requires more land, the Swiss study showed it to be much better for biodiversity, because it "accommodates a greater variety of plants, animals and microorganisms" in and around its fields. Endangered species that are killed off by chemical pesticides can survive under organic systems. Other studies have found that many more birds, insects that birds eat, butterflies, spiders, and earthworms live in or near organic farms. In addition, if we take a long-term view, organic farming's yields will tend to go up over time as scientific knowledge increases while conventional yields may go down as the soil gets depleted and the water runs out.

But this doesn't mean that certified organic agriculture is the best choice in all situations. It will be especially hard in the near term to implement organic methods widely in places like the midwestern corn and wheat belts that are geared around one or two crops. As agricultural economist Rich Welsch points out, "To grow more crops in rotation—a requirement for organic certification—farmers would need to develop an array of new markets and systems for storing and distributing these products."[24] Although a few farmers can develop special niches for themselves, it would require a slow and costly transition to switch most of them over.

Government and consumers should therefore also support farmers who reduce environmental impacts but don't reach organic standards or who incorporate benign practices prohibited by the organic rules, such as the growing of environmentally safe genetically engineered crops. In general, the government should use a combination of incentives and penalties to get farmers to conserve water and soil, to reduce pesticide use, and to make sure that contaminants don't run off the farm into drinking supplies and rivers. Some useful regulations and programs are in place to accomplish these things, but much more needs to be done.

How to Buy Organic

Although it doesn't make sense for all farms to become organic, it is still important for you to support this farming method by buying some organic foods. That is an easy way for you to signal your interest in an environmentally improved food system. There are few comparable labels for other sustainably grown food, so organics are the easiest way to express your preference.

Consumer organic purchases have several indirect benefits. The federal and state governments increased funding for sustainable agriculture research only after politicians and government officials discovered that a significant number of Americans were buying organic foods. And each organic farm has a powerful impact beyond its own borders, by showing other farmers that all those chemicals aren't always necessary. After Fresno, California, farmer John Diener turned 20 percent of his farm into an organic operation with two neighboring farms, he cut his use of commercial phosphate fertilizers by two-thirds on the other 80 percent of his farm, because he had learned that it was possible, practical, and profitable to do so.[25]

Because organic foods cost more than conventional ones, you may want to spend your organic dollars carefully, especially if you are on a tight budget. But it should certainly be worth spending some modest amount extra each week—whether that be $1.00, $5.00, or $10.00—to move our country toward a more environmentally friendly food system. To maximize your health benefit, focus on foods like peaches that conventionally have high pesticide residues (see chapter 4). To buy the most organic food at the least cost, choose organic produce when the price differential is the smallest. When conventional bananas are selling for $0.29 a pound and organic ones are $0.79, you might want to choose the conventional ones. But when the difference in price is only $0.10 or $0.20 a pound, buy organic. If you start looking for organic foods on a regular basis, you will quickly discover which choices make the most sense for you.

But don't use an organic label as an excuse to abandon nutritional sense, especially when it comes to processed foods. Organic potato chips may be just as bad for your health and waistline as any other potato chips. Many organic processed microwave meals have just as much salt, sugar, and fat as conventional ones. So look carefully at the nutrition labels, even when purchasing organic products.

Over time, there are likely to be other useful labels in addition to the organic one. Sustainable farmers who don't meet organic standards will want to distinguish their products from conventional ones, and a few food stores already try to indicate produce that comes from such farms. Food producers who make an extra effort to treat their workers well or to advance social equity will want you to know that as well. As with meat labels, when unknown claims appear on the fruits, vegetables, and grains in your food store, look them up on www.eco-labels.org.

Food You Can Trust

Buying certified organic products is one simple way to find food with smaller environmental impacts, but you can also get your food from identifiable sources that you can learn about and trust. The most certain way is to grow your food yourself using organic, low-impact gardening practices. Many books, magazines, and organizations, some of which we list in the resource guide in Appendix B, can advise you on how to do that. And by planting a vegetable garden or growing fruits, you can take satisfaction from knowing that you are increasing the world's total food supply. If your garden replaces grass, you will also reduce the air pollution and greenhouse gas emissions associated with mowing with a power mower.

You can also get your food at farm stands or farmers' markets where you can actually speak to representatives of the farm to find out about their operations. Between 1994 and 2000, the number of farmers' markets grew by 63 percent. There are now 2,800 across the country, so there is a good chance you can find one near you.[26] But if you can't, you can sometimes get food from local family farms at your neighborhood supermarket.

Oftentimes, buying local has important benefits beyond pollution reduction. In many parts of the country, small-scale farmers face daunting economic challenges and are under pressure to sell their land to developers. If the farms succumb to suburban development, the communities will suffer by becoming more crowded, less interesting, and less diverse. The nation will suffer by losing land for future food production. Buying local foods can be an effective way to help preserve local farmland.

If you do a little investigation, you may find local farms that have laudable practices that go beyond organic. They may, for example, take steps to ensure better conditions for their workers or may encourage worker unions or may participate actively in organizations aimed at helping family farmers. Such exemplary farms certainly deserve your active support.

An innovative way to help worthy local farms is Community Supported Agriculture (CSA). Consumers can become member-subscribers of one of more than 1,000 community-supported farms across the country, promising to pay a periodic fee for regular shipments of fresh produce that vary with the season. The consumers get especially fresh, healthy food and the assurance that they are helping to preserve a valuable local farm; the farmer eliminates the middleman and has the security of having committed buyers. To find out if there are any community-supported farms near you, see the website of the Robyn Van En Center for CSA Resources (www.csacenter.org).

Similarly, small businesses can try negotiating agreements with local farmers to deliver produce to their work sites. Such direct-to-consumer arrangements help farmers by giving them contracts for their produce that more than cover their costs. Organic restaurants sometimes buy a farmer's entire production, even before the first seed is planted.

A DIFFERENT FOOD STORE

Few people would be willing to volunteer hundreds of hours to help the grocery store where they shop, but Marilyn Andrews does just that for Greenfields Market in western Massachusetts. She chairs the board of this food co-op, which has 780 members, as well as several thousand other customers.

Greenfields Market specializes in organic, locally grown, and whole grain foods. Most people who shop there do so because they can choose from a wide range of quality, nonmainstream foods and because they believe the store's management actively screens foods for quality and safety.

Yet it would be unlikely that Andrews and the many other active co-op members would devote so much volunteer time if it were only to be able to get good organic peaches, unusual veggie burgers, or farm-fresh eggs. Because food is so central to people's lives, they have been able to turn the market into one of the town's most important community centers. The friendly atmosphere encourages people to congregate and eat lunch there. A wide range of organizations hold meetings at the market. Co-op members carry out a wide range of projects, including

THE SEAFOOD QUANDARY

So far, we've assessed the impacts of eating meat, dairy, fruits, vegetables, and grains, but how do fish and other seafood stack up? Is it better to eat a tuna steak or a beefsteak? Should you switch from clam chowder to minestrone soup? And when you eat seafood, is it better to choose cod, crab, or calamari?

While we will give you some easy-to-follow recommendations, first we need to admit that it is very hard to make generalizations about the environmental impacts of eating fish. Of the more than three pounds of meat the average American consumes in a week, almost all of it comes from just four animals—cattle, chickens, pigs, and turkeys. In contrast, Americans eat only about a quarter-pound of fish and shellfish each week, yet that includes hundreds of different types, some living in oceans, some in lakes, and some in rivers. Although most fish and shellfish are caught in the wild, a growing proportion of them is raised on fish farms.

---

going into schools to educate young people about nutrition, running a community soup kitchen, and preparing informational pamphlets.

Andrews, a potter by trade, was drawn to join the food co-op when she moved to Massachusetts from Illinois in the mid-1980s, because she saw it as a good way to meet some of her neighbors and become involved in the community. When she discovered that the co-op was overtaxing the most involved members so much that it risked falling apart, she was one of the people who decided to put more energy into it to make sure it survived and grew. "We needed to give a lot of attention to group process," Andrews recalls, "not only so we could make some difficult decisions but to build trust and so that co-op members would feel good about the time they spent helping the market."

For Andrews, the most satisfying payback is that the many people who now shop at Greenfields Market get to see and experience an alternative model of a business. "By its continued existence," Andrews notes, "Greenfields Market raises for people the possibility that our society can do things differently. You can have different institutions than the usual corporate for-profit ones—ones that people can trust and that build community."

Even within a specific type of fish or shellfish there is often tremendous variety. For example, there are cherrystone clams, littleneck clams, and long-neck clams. There are Atlantic salmon and Pacific salmon. Among Pacific salmon, there are five major species and several hundred substocks ranging from pink salmon, which weigh about 3.5 to 4 pounds, to chinook salmon, which frequently grow to more than 30 pounds.

Given this rich diversity, it is impossible to make blanket statements about whether it is better or worse for the environment to eat fish or meat, for instance. There are considerable differences in the environmental impacts associated with eating different types of fish. Before explaining your options at the grocery store or restaurant, here's a brief analysis of the three main environmental problems caused by eating fish.

1. Eating a Particular Fish or Shellfish Can Wipe Out That Species

Fishing fleets have been catching so many fish that they have depleted the number living in many locations. Modern technology has made it possible to gather fish ever more efficiently. Globally, we harvest six times more ocean fish than in 1950. The Food and Agriculture Organization (FAO) of the United Nations estimates that about half of the world's stocks of ocean fish are fully exploited; any additional fishing would cause the fish populations to decline. More troubling, an additional 15 to 18 percent of fish stocks are already overexploited and will continue to decline unless strong action is taken to end excessive fishing. Close to home, the U.S. National Marine Fisheries Service reports that 100 out of the 300 U.S. fisheries for which there is data are either overfished (i.e., being fished faster than the fish can reproduce) or close to it.[27]

Here are two examples of dramatic fish declines caused in great part by overfishing: First, between 1975 and 2000, the number of adult Atlantic salmon returning to North American rivers fell from 1.5 million a year to less than a quarter that number. And second, the average size of the swordfish that commercial fishing vessels caught in the North Atlantic fell from 266 pounds in 1963 to 90 pounds in 1995. Because female swordfish don't breed until they are five years old and weigh 150 pounds, fishing eliminated many young swordfish before they could reproduce.[28]

Perhaps the saddest and most dramatic collapse of a fish species took place in what had once been one of the world's most amazing treasure troves of fish—the Grand Banks region off Newfoundland. Back in the seventeenth century, there were so many cod that English sailors reported "that we heardlie have been able to row a boate through them."[29] Over several hundred years, heavy fishing first gradually and then rapidly depleted the stock. Then, starting in the 1950s, huge 400-foot factory-freezer trawlers from around the world began to scoop up cod in astounding quantities, each processing more than 650 tons of fish daily.[30] Although government officials in Canada could have predicted the inevitable outcome, they were slow to react. By the late 1980s, the fishery was collapsing and many Newfoundland fishers were out of work. By 1992, when the Canadian government belatedly closed the Grand Banks to fishing, scientists estimated that there were only a little more than 1 percent of the number of adult cod in the area as there had been 30 years earlier![31] And even though fishing has now stopped, some scientists believe that the mix of animals and plants in the area has been so changed by decades of intensive fishing that the cod population may never revive.

Overfishing is often a classic case of what ecologist Garret Hardin called "the tragedy of the commons."[32] In his model, the oceans are like a common pasture, where each individual has an economic incentive to use the common resource as much as possible. Unilateral action to use less only hurts the individual, because someone else would take whatever was left behind. Over time, all those economically rational individual actions end up devastating the commons, robbing future generations of a valuable resource.

It's important to step back and realize what overfishing destroys. Not only are humans decimating complex, rich, wonderful ecosystems filled with diverse plants and animals, but we are reducing our ability to provide adequate nourishment to a growing world population. Fish and shellfish provide one-sixth of the animal protein that humans consume worldwide.[33] Moreover, a billion people get most of their animal protein from fish. And those in many poorer countries, including Bangladesh, Congo, Ghana, Indonesia, and North Korea, rely heavily on fish for protein.

To end the "tragedy of the commons" at sea, governments need to impose strong rules that restrict how many fish are captured. Some useful steps have been taken in places such as Georges Bank off Cape Cod, but mostly it has been too little and too late. And even when sound restrictions are put in place, they can be hard to enforce, since they often involve keeping track of hard-to-monitor limits on the size of fishing nets or the number of crew members or the total weight of a boat's catch.

To get around this problem, scientists, including the authoritative National Academy of Sciences (NAS), have increasingly advocated the creation of marine reserves—areas of the ocean where fishing is totally banned. Using global positioning satellites (GPSs), governments can easily track whether vessels enter the reserves, although they also need to maintain patrols to catch poachers who don't agree to participate in GPS tracking. A recent study by the National Center for Ecological Analysis and Synthesis found that within two years of the establishment of this type of reserve, the number of fish increases an average of 91 percent while fish size increases 31 percent. These safe havens, where small fish can grow to maturity, not only increase fish stocks within their boundaries but in nearby waters as well, thus providing important benefits to the fishing industry. In 2000 and 2001, the U.S. government and the state of Florida set aside the nation's largest ocean refuge—the Tortugas Ecological Reserve, an area of 151 square nautical miles off the Florida Keys.[34]

But marine reserves alone will not solve overfishing. There needs to be greater communication and new sorts of cooperative efforts among scientists, fishers, and government regulators to come up with innovative protection strategies for fisheries. Up to now, each group has tended to view the others as naive and uninformed. Fishers experience the day-to-day reality of life on the sea. As Maryland waterman Bill Clayton dismissively points out, "We look at that water daily; the college-degree people go by things they learned in books."[35] For their part, the scientists think many fishers are blinded by their immediate economic needs and cultural traditions and don't always understand the complex relationships among the many species in marine habitats. Scientists and fishers both can find government officials to be mindless, arbitrary bureaucrats. In reality, each of the three groups has unique knowledge that is essential to crafting the best solutions. Moreover, fishers will be less likely to look for ways to skirt government regulations if they are involved in establishing those regulations.

At the consumption level, retailers, restaurants, and consumers can help stop overfishing by avoiding certain types of fish. A boycott of Atlantic swordfish after 1997 by environmental groups and many individual Americans reduced sales, focused attention on a serious problem, and helped bring about an international recovery plan.

2. Eating Fish or Shellfish Can Wipe Out Other Species

This second problem relates to overfishing, but often represents even more thoughtless and shortsighted behavior. Many modern fishing vessels are designed to capture one or two particular types of fish. The boat owners often find it cost-effective to throw out any other types of fish that accidentally get caught in their nets. This so-called bycatch can be huge—about one-quarter of all the ocean fish caught by weight.[36] Unfortunately, the bycatch dies in the process—a stunningly wasteful enterprise.

Shrimp fishing is especially problematic. Although a growing percentage of shrimp in American restaurants and supermarkets comes from fish farms (and this, as we will see, has its own problems), almost half is still caught in the wild. Sadly, when fishing for shrimp, the usable shrimp may only be one-sixth of the total catch and the remaining bycatch is wasted.[37] The dragnet used in shrimp fishing can convert a rich aquatic environment into a virtual moonscape.

Besides bycatch, there is another way in which eating fish or shellfish can wipe out other species. As demand for fish increases and the stock of some of the larger species, such as cod and swordfish, declines, fishing fleets and consumers shift to smaller types of fish, ones farther down the food chain.[38] As this happens, few people consider the impact on the larger fish that would normally feed on the small fry. In one extreme case, Soviet fishing vessels entered the Grand Banks in the 1970s to catch capelin, a tiny smeltlike fish. The Canadian government gave the Soviets its blessing even though capelin were the cod's favorite food. After three years of overfishing, the capelin had been nearly wiped out, making it much more difficult for the cod to survive. Similarly, heavy fishing of capelin, sand eel, and Norway pout in the North Sea helped lead to the decline of cod, seals, and seabirds.[39]

The recent increase in aquaculture (fish farming) could accelerate the decline of small feeder-fish species. At most salmon and shrimp farms, the feed includes fish meal. Large quantities of anchovies, herring, mackerel, sardines, and other small fish are captured and ground up into fish meal for use in aquaculture. In fact, the farms use two to five times more fish protein than they produce. This hasn't caused serious new problems yet because most of the fish meal has been diverted from other uses in animal agriculture.[40] But as fish farming continues to expand, this practice could deplete valuable species. This problem could be minimized by focusing fish farming on plant-eating species such as catfish, mussels, and tilapia, and by developing new feeds for those species that normally eat fish. This is only one of several important reasons for carefully regulating fish farming.

3. Eating Fish or Shellfish Can Pollute and Destroy Valuable Habitats

Both fish farming and ocean fishing can cause significant environmental damage. At first glance, fish farming might seem like a completely benign, positive solution to overfishing and the collapse of so many fisheries. Already more than a quarter of the fish produced for human uses worldwide comes from fish farms, and this number will continue to rise rapidly.[41] Yet fish farming can actually increase pollution and damage essential natural ecosystems.

As with everything related to fish, it's hard to make blanket generalizations about fish farming, since it is practiced in many different places in many different ways. China has practiced aquaculture for thousands of years and now raises more fish and shellfish than the rest of the world combined. India, Japan, and other Asian nations are the next biggest fish farmers, but the United States, Europe, and other parts of the world are rapidly expanding their production. The biggest Asian products are carp and clams and other mollusks. Americans primarily eat farmed shrimp, catfish, salmon, and trout.

Crawfish and clam farming causes fewer problems than shrimp farming. Salmon farms in Maine do less environmental harm than those in Scotland. Some of the shrimp farms in Thailand are much more sustainably managed than others in the same country.

In general, it is important to remember that most fish farms are not isolated from the wider ocean or lake environment. Diseases frequently develop in the crowded conditions of fish farms and then spread to wild relatives, decimating their numbers. Fish farms also often experience escapes. In just one instance, a storm off Stone Island, Maine, damaged a fish farm's steel-cage system, permitting 100,000 salmon to get out. The escaped fish can take over the habitats of indigenous species or can breed with natives, making the resulting offspring less able to survive in the wild. In British Columbia, for example, an average of more than 40,000 farm-raised Atlantic salmon have escaped each year since 1994, and some of them have invaded the spawning territory of threatened Pacific salmon species.[42]

Some fish farms pollute coastal areas by adding antibiotics to the water or discharging large quantities of fish meal and waste. If the farm is in a location where tides frequently exchange the water, this may not be a problem, but fish farms have not always been carefully located. In Scotland, for example, salmon farms located at the relatively stagnant heads of sea lochs can produce as much waste as the sewage from 20,000 people. Glasgow University biologist Colin Adams notes that "in the deep, glacial lochs around the farms the flushing rate is so poor that it is akin to flushing your toilet once every two weeks." The excess nutrients in the water helped close down some of the area's shellfish fisheries by spawning toxic algae blooms, which can cause severe neurological problems.[43]

Many people around the world have been especially critical of shrimp farming.[44] And indeed, the industry's rapid expansion in the 1980s and 1990s was poorly planned. Some farms were placed in unworkable locations where they soon had to be abandoned. Others in developing countries destroyed fishing grounds for subsistence fishers. Perhaps most tragically, some shrimp-farm developers destroyed valuable mangrove trees, especially in Southeast Asia. Mangroves not only serve as protective nurseries for various commercially important fish species, but they provide firewood for local residents and soak up excess nutrients that would otherwise pollute the water. Cutting down the mangroves caused erosion, which clogged the water with soil, smothering the living corals that make up nearby coral reefs. Although shrimp farming wasn't the major cause of mangrove destruction, it was an important contributing factor. A series of international meetings eliminated the most egregious practices, but most shrimp farming remains problematic.

So, all in all, aquaculture is not a panacea. Yet on balance it can play a positive role in global food supply as long as the siting and operation of fish farms are more carefully regulated than in the past. Citizens, especially those who live in states with fish farms, like Maine, can speak up in support of putting aquaculture on a more sustainable basis.

Fishing, as opposed to aquaculture, is far from blameless when it comes to pollution and destruction of habitats. Bottom trawling, which involves dragging heavy nets across the seafloor, has been especially damaging to plants, animals, and the physical features of the ocean bottom. As ecologist Peter Auster notes, "The nets are held open by heavy doors called otter boards that can weigh up to a ton. The leading edge of the net itself usually has chains or metal bobbins weighing tens to hundreds of pounds each to force fish or shrimp to rise off the seafloor and get caught in the net."[45] Anything in the way—coral, sponges, anemones, shell beds, worms, rocks—is plowed over and flattened. Fishing vessels that dredge for mussels, oysters, and scallops can have a similar effect.

To monitor the impact, Auster dove underwater and actually "sat on the seafloor and watched a scallop dredge ramble by, and then swam into the path where the dredge had just passed to see much of the complexity of the seafloor removed; what was once a complex of sponges, shells, and other organisms was smoothed to a cobblestone street."[46]

In a widely quoted article, prominent marine scientists Les Watling and Elliott Norse compared bottom trawling to the clear-cutting of forests. Except bottom trawling takes place on a much wider scale—150 times the area of forest clear-cutting, or several million square miles per year. Once the trawlers pass by, it can take years, decades, or even centuries for the habitat to recover. Some places are trawled hundreds of times a year. Not only are remarkable environments harmed and marine creatures killed, but the fish supply goes down, since many baby fish rely on the hiding places that a complex, unsmoothed seafloor provides.[47] And in recent years, new technologies have allowed trawling on rocky ocean bottoms that used to be inaccessible.

But because the trawling takes place away from the public's gaze, it gets much less attention than forest clear-cutting. Watling observes that "if 300-year-old redwoods were being cut along the coast of California to make way for agricultural crops, there would be hell to pay. Yet, equivalent actions are occurring daily under the sea. . . . Fishermen operate out of sight of nearly everyone, and because of that, levels of environmental destruction that would be prohibited outright on land are routine."[48]

Many of the solutions to overfishing, such as marine reserves and fishing limits, would also protect parts of the seafloor from trawling. In addition, governments could regulate the types of trawling and dredging equipment that is used in particularly valuable locations.

What You Can Do to Protect Fish and Oceans

Clearly, many fish species are in trouble and humans are destroying valuable ocean habitats. But what exactly should we do about it when we shop or eat out?

It would be extremely helpful if there were an easy way to distinguish fish that had been caught or farmed in a sustainable manner from more problematic choices. Unfortunately, there is currently nothing comparable to the organic label for fruits, vegetables, grains, and meats, although various organizations are trying to move things in this direction. The international Marine Stewardship Council has been working on the most extensive fish-labeling initiative. The environmental group World Wildlife Fund (WWF) and Unilever (one of the world's largest fish buyers) initially sponsored that council, but it is now an independent nonprofit organization. The quantity of fish receiving the council's seal of approval remains small but should grow in the future. In September 2000, Alaskan wild salmon became the first fish from American waters to receive council certification.

In addition, several private businesses and business associations have begun to specialize in environmentally friendly seafood. Ecofish sells sustainably caught fish, including some with Marine Stewardship Council certification, to restaurants and natural food stores nationwide. The Cape Cod Commercial Hook Fishermen's Association works with New England fishers to promote fish caught using environmentally sound methods, such as fishing with hooks rather than nets.

Ultimately, a good labeling system is the only thing that can provide consumers with an easy way to distinguish among all the dozens of different types of fish available. For that reason, the most important and most useful action you can take is to support the nascent labeling efforts by purchasing fish certified by the Marine Stewardship Council or sold by one of the sustainability-oriented businesses. Also ask your local food stores and restaurants to carry certified sustainable seafood and buy it if they stock it. By taking these steps, you will ensure that consumers in the future have simple guidance for making environmentally sound seafood choices.

While a widespread labeling system will take years to establish, in the meantime, four knowledgeable organizations—Environmental Defense, the Monterey Bay Aquarium, the National Audubon Society, and the Natural Resources Defense Council—have placed lists of good and problematic seafood on their websites.[49] The National Audubon Society has also produced the *Seafood Lover's Almanac,* a handsome illustrated book that shows what different fish look like, explains how they are caught or farmed, and rates whether they are wise consumer choices or not.[50] Although the four organizations generally agree on their recommendations, they don't all cover the same fish and a few of their conclusions are different. Moreover, as some fisheries improve while others decline, the lists change to reflect the most current information.

Although some of the groups offer handy wallet-sized cards summarizing their recommendations, most consumers won't want to try to keep track of 40 or 50 different seafood types when they go to the grocery store or out to eat. A simpler, more practical approach is to remember just a few of the best and a few of the worst. Avoid the latter and try to buy the former. Pay less attention to the large number of other types between the best and the worst, and make your choices among those on taste, nutrition, price, and other grounds other than the environment.

The short list of fish and shellfish to remember uses the consensus choices of the four organizations. The chart below lists seafood types that the organizations agree on and which at least three of the four evaluate. Other types of seafood may be equally good or bad, but there's not the same strong expert consensus about them.

FISH AND SHELLFISH TO REMEMBER

Good choices	Bad choices
Alaskan salmon	Atlantic swordfish
Catfish	Chilean sea bass (Patagonian toothfish)
Mahimahi (dolphinfish)	Cod
Pacific Dungeness crab	Orange roughy
Pacific halibut	Pacific rockfish (rock cod)
Striped bass	Red snapper
Tilapia	Shark

As a final useful strategy for exercising your consumer power, ask lots of questions at food stores and restaurants about the fish they sell. This will expand your knowledge and show them that they have alert, concerned customers. Mark Kurlansky, author of the book *Cod: A Biography of the Fish That Changed the World,* asks us to remember that most fish for sale are wild animals. If you "went into a store and there were rhinoceros steaks and some tiger chops, you'd ask a few questions. When you go into a fish store and you see some new species you've never heard of before . . . you should be asking where does it come from and how is it caught. You'll usually find that the fish merchant won't be able to answer the question but if people keep asking these questions [knowing the answers] will become a part of running a fish store."[51] Ultimately, selling fish caught or raised in environmentally sound ways will become an important marketing tool for seafood merchants.

CHAPTER FOUR

PESTICIDES AND CHEMICALS IN THE FOOD SUPPLY

Conventionally grown foods, including fruits, vegetables, grains, and even meat, can contain trace amounts of toxic chemicals and pesticide residues. While the presence of these chemicals doesn't necessarily make your food unsafe (and in fact the food industry says they pose little or no danger at all), there are few scientific studies documenting the long-term consequences of this chemical exposure. In 1987 the Environmental Protection Agency (EPA) estimated that pesticide residues on food might cause cancer in as many as 6,000 people annually in the United States.[1] For the individual consumer, that risk may seem small. But it certainly isn't small if it is your family member who faces chemotherapy or the cloud of living with cancer.

Even though pesticides and other chemicals in our food are a public health concern, the risks should not discourage you from eating plenty of fruits and vegetables. In fact, it would be worse for your overall health to stop eating fruits and vegetables to avoid pesticide residues than to keep eating them, pesticides and all. Luckily, it isn't an either/or choice. You can intelligently reduce the amount of pesticides and other chemicals you eat while maintaining a diet with a rich variety of fresh fruits and vegetables. This chapter will tell you how.

Unlike the effects of harmful bacteria in food, which are usually apparent within a few hours or days of eating the food, the health effects caused by pesticides and other chemicals in our diets are far removed from the act of eating. Cancer and other chronic effects may not occur for years or even decades after the toxic chemicals in food have been consumed.

PESTICIDES: THE ALAR STORY

In the decades following World War II, pesticides provided the same type of revolution for farming that antibiotics provided for medicine. Suddenly farmers had tools to control hazards—like insect pests, weeds, and plant viruses—that killed their crops or reduced their yields. Pesticides dramatically increased the amount of food and other crops farmers could produce while reducing the amount of farmland needed to grow the crops. But the change was not entirely benign.

If the impact of pesticide use had been limited to insect, viral, and plant pests, then the story would end on the farm, a tale of human ingenuity overcoming adversity. But in order to be effective, the chemicals used to treat plants had to be toxic. Unfortunately, sometimes that toxicity extended to humans as well.

The government has played an active role in approving and monitoring the use of pesticides and other agricultural chemicals, including, for the last 50 years, setting maximum levels of pesticide residues in food. Many of these government-established pesticide "tolerances," however, don't reflect modern safety standards. The Food Quality Protection Act, a food-safety law enacted in 1996, reduced some of the risks to consumers. But there is still a long way to go.

Another way to reduce risks posed by pesticides is to increase consumers' choice through pesticide labeling. In fact, there is widespread public support for such labeling. In an opinion poll taken in 2001 by the Center for Science in the Public Interest (CSPI), 76 percent of consumers said they wanted food sprayed with pesticides to be labeled.[2] However, today labels don't list the pesticides in food, which means consumers have no way of knowing whether, what, and how much of a pesticide is on their food.

The fear of unknown effects from pesticides in food can impact consumer buying behavior. That was dramatically illustrated when consumers stopped purchasing apples after the nonprofit Natural Resources Defense Council disclosed that certain apples were treated with a potentially carcinogenic plant-growth regulator called Alar. Alar, the trade name for daminozide, was used to improve the quality of red apples and other fruits by increasing their firmness, color, and storage time. Scientists had known since the 1970s that a breakdown product of Alar caused cancer in animal studies and the EPA had twice tried to ban it, unsuccessfully. The agency was hamstrung by a weak law and could not halt the chemical's use. When the agency's impotence came to light nearly 10 years later, the reaction was dramatic.[3]

In February 1989, a CBS *60 Minutes* segment called " 'A' Is for Apple" featured the connection between Alar and cancerous tumors in lab rodents. Ed Bradley opened the segment by saying, "The most potent cancer-causing agent in our food supply is a substance sprayed on apples to keep them on the trees longer and make them look better."[4] The program went on to discuss children's susceptibility to Alar and its by-products. Prior to this *60 Minutes* show, few consumers were aware that food-safety regulations were not sufficient to protect children from harmful pesticides.

The public reacted strongly after the program aired. People discarded apples and refused to buy any that they thought might contain the pesticide. School districts from Los Angeles to New York took apples, applesauce, and apple juice off their menus until further investigations could be completed. Many industry officials have complained that the media reports on Alar were alarmist, and that the apple industry, especially in Washington State, suffered millions of dollars in losses. A few companies had anticipated the public concern. Some, like Gerber and the makers of Mott's apple products, had already stopped using fruits treated with Alar.[5]

Following this episode, apple growers discontinued using Alar and apple sales rebounded. However, Alar provided both the government and the food industry with an important reminder: Consumers vote with their wallets every time they go to the grocery store. If consumers lose confidence in the safety of a particular product, they stop buying it. It is a lesson that is repeated over and over again, whenever there is a major food scare.

Alar provided an American preview for what happened in Europe following the discoveries about the link between BSE (mad cow disease) and human illness, when consumer confidence in both the meat industry and many European governments hit rock bottom. In addition, the Alar episode demonstrated that strong government programs help protect the food industry from scares like Alar. When gaps in regulation or inadequate enforcement of laws allow unsafe foods on the market, strong actions must be taken to revive consumer confidence.

BETTER LIVING THROUGH CHEMISTRY

Romantic visions of farming are commonplace. They persist in children's storybooks and in the minds of many city dwellers. We imagine family farms that raise many diverse crops and animals. In fact, that is what most farming looked like prior to World War II. Farmers controlled their pests through crop rotation and cultivation, grew forage for their animals, and returned animal manure to the land. There was little use of pesticides in those days, and the ones that were used were frequently developed by the farmers themselves, through trial and error.[6]

Today, U.S. farmers produce much of our food on huge tracts that grow one or just a few crops. Many animals raised for meat spend their whole life in confinement systems, where every part of their growth is monitored and controlled. And agriculture is the single heaviest user of pesticides.[7]

After World War II, farmers' use of pesticides grew. The total production of synthetic pesticides in the United States increased tenfold, from 124 million pounds in 1947 to 1.3 billion pounds of active pesticide ingredients in 1997. That is a staggering quantity of toxic material to be spreading on fields, lawns, and gardens. In addition, virtually all pesticides contain so-called inert ingredients, which don't include the active pesticide agent, but are used for storage or application purposes. These inert ingredients, many of which are toxic, can make up 90 percent or more of the contents of the pesticide bag. In 1998, the EPA identified over 50 substances of toxicological concern among the "inert" ingredients used in pesticides, and at least 21 of the "inert" ingredients have been classified as carcinogens.[8]

Decades of carte-blanche use of pesticides and fertilizers have taken a serious toll on water quality, food safety, public health, and fish and wildlife habitat in the United States. The potential side effects of heavy chemical use in agriculture, in homes and offices, and on lawns and gardens were not adequately recognized and considered from the outset. Although a few scientists, such as Rachel Carson, raised serious questions about the potential health effects posed by pesticides, their concerns were often dismissed as "hysterical" reactions to the new wave of technology symbolized by DuPont's corporate slogan: "Better Living Through Chemistry."[9]

Over the past 50 years, researchers have been identifying and quantifying the damage caused by the extensive use of pesticides. In many instances, the full extent of the problem will not be known for years. What is clear, though, is that this national problem is enormous, has many facets, and will require substantial changes in farming practices and consumer habits to effectively reduce future damage.[10]

Experts estimate that the indirect costs of pesticide use may now approach $13.3 billion annually, including over $8.3 billion spent on public health and environmental problems. Those costs include immediate health effects such as human pesticide poisonings and chronic health problems such as cancer. Environmental effects include groundwater contamination, animal pesticide poisonings, reduced natural enemies, pesticide resistance, honeybee poisonings and reduced pollination, losses of crops and trees, and fishery and wildlife losses.[11]

CATCH-22: INSECTS AND WEEDS ADAPT TO PESTICIDE USE

Ironically, American farming's widespread use of pesticides since World War II has not eliminated or necessarily reduced pest problems. The more pesticides are used, the greater the likelihood that the target insects and other pests will develop a natural resistance to the chemicals. This can create a vicious cycle of increasing pesticide use even as the pesticides become less and less effective. In some cases, more expensive, toxic, or ecologically hazardous pesticides must be used.

There are three reasons pesticides stop working. First, the pests that are targeted by a pesticide may develop a resistance to it. Second, the targeted pests can return after the pesticide treatment is over. Finally, the elimination of one pest can create an opportunity for other pests to invade the field, thereby necessitating larger and more frequent applications of pesticides.

For similar reasons, widespread use of herbicides stimulates weeds to develop resistance to those herbicides. In fact, over the past 10 years, the number of weed species resistant to herbicides multiplied more than five times, increasing from 48 to 270.[12]

USING PESTICIDES: TODAY AND IN THE FUTURE

Altogether, according to the EPA, over 20,000 pesticide products are approved for use in the United States. They can be divided into three types: herbicides, which target plant pests; insecticides, which target insects; and fungicides, which target fungal pests. Herbicides are applied to about half of all cropland, with 90 percent of herbicide applications being applied to just four crops: corn, soybeans, cotton, and wheat.[13]

Fruits and vegetables receive the highest application of insecticides and fungicides. Pesticide use varies widely by region. Florida, California, Arizona, and Georgia use the most agricultural chemicals per acre for almost all categories, including both pesticides and fertilizers.[14]

The Food and Drug Administration (FDA) and the U.S. Department of Agriculture (USDA) each run programs that monitor the levels of pesticides in the food supply by testing individual food samples. These programs provide important information about pesticides in our diets. By 1999, about 40 percent of the domestic food samples analyzed by the FDA contained detectable levels of pesticide residues. However, the vast majority of these had residues within the EPA's human tolerance levels. Of the imported food sampled by the FDA, the results were similar.[15]

While these sampling programs are informative, they suffer from critical weaknesses. For one thing, each year the FDA samples less than one-half of 1 percent of the more than 4 million food shipments that are imported into the United States (mainly fruits and vegetables). Moreover, 3.7 percent of domestic samples and 3 percent of the imported ones contain pesticide residues for which the government agencies have no legal tolerance. That means we're eating a lot of food that simply should not be on the market. And the FDA's routine lab methods can detect only half of the pesticides applied to food, which means that the agency's results may grossly underestimate the actual amount of pesticides in food.[16]

Furthermore, the FDA does not test a representative sample of what people eat. Additional information available from the USDA's testing of fruits and vegetables shows that there are some foods especially popular with children, like apples and strawberries, that contain one or more pesticide residues in over 95 percent of the samples.

Government monitoring for pesticide residues in food gives us both bad news and good news: A large amount of food is contaminated, but with very low levels of pesticides. If government pesticide tolerances adequately protected human health, then these results could be considered mostly good news. Unfortunately, the Alar episode demonstrated that pesticide standards set by the government are not always adequate to safeguard children and other vulnerable consumers.

How consumers are affected by ongoing exposure to pesticide residues remains unclear. In part because it is unethical to test toxic pesticides on people, no definitive research studies have linked pesticide residues in food to human illnesses. Although many pesticides may be harmless, scientists think residues of some pesticides increase the risk of cancer and noncancerous tumors, disruption of the endocrine system, allergic reactions, and a syndrome known as multiple chemical sensitivity.[17]

Acute toxic reactions to pesticide residues on food are easier to trace than chronic conditions, but are rare. In a noteworthy 1985 case, 1,000 people were poisoned in several western states and Canada after eating watermelons that had been illegally treated with the insecticide aldicarb. Within hours after eating the watermelon, the victims experienced nausea, vomiting, blurred vision, muscle weakness, and other symptoms. Estimates of the doses that caused the illnesses were well below the laboratory detection limit, a supposedly safe level.[18]

Farmers, farmworkers, and others in farm communities have the greatest contact with pesticides—both directly on the farm and through their drinking water, which tends to be more contaminated than water at a greater distance from agricultural areas. It is not surprising that they suffer more health problems from pesticides than the rest of the population. A 1992 review by the National Cancer Institute of approximately two dozen reports concluded that farmers had increased risks of such forms of cancer as Hodgkin's disease, multiple myeloma, leukemia, melanoma, and cancers of the lip, prostate, and stomach. Pesticide exposure was named as one of the key causes of these cancers. The farmers otherwise had lower rates of mortality from heart disease and certain other cancers (lung, esophagus, bladder, colon, liver, and kidney) than the rest of the population, possibly because of low prevalence of smoking, low body fat, or high levels of physical activity.[19]

POISONED: A STORY OF FARMWORKERS

In 1993, Phosdrin, an extremely toxic pesticide, was used to kill aphids in the apple orchards in Washington State. It was substituted for another, safer pesticide after that pesticide's registration was not renewed by the manufacturer. Phosdrin emerged as the only substitute that didn't lead to insect resistance. Although Phosdrin is more toxic than many other pesticides used in the orchards, Washington State put no restrictions on who could mix and load it.

Phosdrin was linked to 27 farmworker poisoning cases in Washington that year. Twenty-three workers were exposed during preparation and application of the pesticide, while three were exposed to the residues (the final poisoned farmworker didn't participate in the follow-up study). These farmworkers went to hospital emergency rooms around the state with poisoning symptoms, including headaches, wheezing, nausea, convulsions, and paralysis. Experts reviewing the situation believe that many other poisoning cases went unreported. Following this incident, Washington State banned the use of Phosdrin in the apple orchards.

Sources: Hugo Flores et al., *The Phosdrin Lesson* (Olympia, Wash.: Evergreen State College, 1994); Occupational Safety and Health Administration, "Chemical Sampling Information," rev. January 12, 1999, available at www.osha-slc.gov/dts/chemicalsampling/data/CH_262100.html.

USE AND MISUSE OF PESTICIDES:
THE LEGAL FRAMEWORK

Three federal agencies have joint responsibility for regulating pesticides. The EPA approves the use of pesticides when evidence shows that they will not cause unreasonable risk to human health and the environment. The EPA also sets the maximum amount, or "tolerance," of a pesticide residue that is allowed in or on a food. The FDA and the USDA then jointly enforce the tolerances set by the EPA on all domestic and imported foods.[20]

Pesticide laws were first developed following World War II. From the very beginning, Congress chose to treat pesticides used in farming differently from food additives in processed foods. This difference was largely due to the fact that Congress believed that pesticides had greater importance for providing an adequate and economical food supply. The laws governing pesticides and food additives were both enacted in the 1950s, but until recently they utilized very different legal approaches to protect the public.[21]

Food additives are used in processed food to improve their color and texture or to extend their shelf life. These chemicals are approved by the Food and Drug Administration, following a review of the manufacturer's research. A new additive must pose a "reasonable certainty of no harm" to consumers. Because of this, most food additives are safe, although there have been some exceptions.

In contrast, the EPA sets pesticide tolerances only after giving consideration to the value of each particular chemical to producing "an adequate and wholesome food supply." That approach, in which risks to consumers were weighed against production benefits, was built into the statutory requirements in the 1950s.

An additional requirement applied to both food additives and pesticides if they caused cancer. An amendment to the food-additive law, called the Delaney clause, stated that chemicals that caused cancer were prohibited in processed foods. This "zero tolerance" also applied to cancer-causing pesticides that became more concentrated during processing.[22]

Despite these legal standards and protections, pesticides with the potential to cause serious public health effects still entered the food sup-ply. In part, they slipped through legal loopholes in the original law. For example, some highly toxic chemicals were "grandfathered" under the 1954 Pesticide Act. In addition, the ban on carcinogenic chemicals in food implemented through the Delaney clause did not apply to chemicals used exclusively on raw agricultural products. Thus, the Delaney clause did not fully protect consumers. It did minimize the risk of carcinogens in processed foods, but it allowed residues of cancer-causing chemicals on unprocessed foods.[23]

There were other glaring problems with pesticide regulation under the old laws. The EPA and the FDA regulated pesticides individually, which failed to account for cumulative effects of exposure to several pesticides. But food frequently contains more than one pesticide. For example, in one study researchers found 10 different pesticides in two apple samples, 12 different pesticides in two orange samples, and 11 different pesticides in one pear sample. If the pesticides exhibit a com-mon toxicity, then the combined effect could be serious.[24] But the com-bined effects of multiple exposures was never considered in setting tolerances.

In the late 1980s and early 1990s, three things happened that set the stage for rewriting the standards for regulating pesticides in food. First, in 1987, the Delaney clause was the subject of a National Academy of Sciences (NAS) report with the intriguing subtitle *The Delaney Paradox*. In this report, experts found that there was no "scientific or policy reason for regulating pesticides present in or on raw commodities differently than those present on processed food." The committee continued: "From the standpoint of consumer protection, the source of exposure—raw commodity versus processed food—seems irrelevant. The other incon-sistency is the system's disparate treatment of old and new pesticides. Old pesticides, especially those first registered before 1972, generally were not tested adequately."[25]

The EPA partially addressed these problems by not fully en-forcing the Delaney clause. In 1988, the agency announced a policy that permitted concentrations of cancer-causing pesticide residues in processed foods above the Delaney "zero tolerance" if the pesticide posed only a "de minimis" risk of causing cancer. This allowed the

EPA to approve several pesticides that posed an estimated cancer risk of 1 in 1 million, rather than the zero-tolerance standard mandated by the Delaney clause.[26]

The Natural Resources Defense Council (NRDC) and other groups challenged this new policy and petitioned the EPA to fully enforce the Delaney clause. When the EPA denied the petition, the environmental groups sued the EPA. Over the next five years, environmental groups battled the government in the courts. The court of appeals ultimately agreed with the NRDC, stating that "the language is clear and mandatory. The Delaney clause provides that no additive shall be deemed safe if it induces cancer. . . . The statute provides that once the finding of carcinogenicity is made, the EPA has no discretion." The decision continued: "The EPA in effect asks us to approve what it deems to be a more

---

STRAWBERRIES WITHOUT PESTICIDES

In 1983, when Jim Cochran decided to experiment by becoming the first California farmer to grow strawberries without using chemical pesticides, his neighbors thought he was doomed to failure. As Cochran acknowledged, "Growing strawberries is a real high-stakes game," costing $30,000 per acre to produce. If a grower makes a mistake, it costs 10 times more than a mistake with a simpler crop like broccoli. "So it's real nerve-wracking."*

Why, then, did Cochran choose to forgo the use of pesticides? After all, more than most crops, strawberries are vulnerable to insects and hard-to-control weeds. But Cochran had discovered what pesticides can do to farmers, farmworkers, and others who come in contact with them. He wanted to try a different approach.

He especially wanted to eliminate the use of methyl bromide, a highly toxic pesticide that scientists now know has the added disadvantage of harming the ozone layer. Farmers fumigate their strawberry fields with this chemical to control weeds, diseases, parasites, and insects in the soil. Methyl bromide treatments allow continuous strawberry production in the same field year after year.

* Quoted in "Why Organic Berries Cost So Much," *Farmers Market Outlook* (May 1996), p. 3.

enlightened system than that which Congress established. The EPA is not alone in criticizing the scheme established by the Delaney clause. . . . Revising the existing statutory scheme, however, is neither our function nor the function of the EPA."[27]

The court affirmed that regardless of the value of the Delaney clause as public policy, it was the law of the land until Congress changed it. The EPA could not act unilaterally. This decision was the second major event that made enactment of the new law inevitable.

The third and final event occurred a few months later, when the NAS released another report, *Pesticides in the Diets of Infants and Children.* This study found additional weaknesses in the structure for regulating pesticides. In part a response to the Alar scare, an expert group formed by the NAS found that pesticide tolerances

---

"The experts said you could never get a crop without them," Cochran recalls. "Disproving them became an obsession with me."**

Over several years, he switched his Swanton Berry Farms to pesticide-free organic methods and worked with an entomologist at the University of California, Santa Cruz to develop chemical-free pest-control techniques. Because he has to rotate his strawberries with other crops and requires extra labor, his costs are higher. They are also higher because he pays higher wages than most strawberry growers, being the first to sign a contract with the United Farm Workers. But through direct marketing to stores and consumers, as well as increased interest in organic produce, he receives higher prices for his fruit.

Nearly 20 years after he began to abandon pesticides, Jim Cochran appears farsighted rather than foolhardy. He has a step up on other farmers, especially now that the EPA is phasing out methyl bromide by 2005. Cochran's success has encouraged other strawberry farmers to try organic methods, and more than 2 percent of the strawberries grown are now organic. Even those farmers who continue to use pesticides can see that chemicals are not as essential as they once thought and are finding ways to cut down.

** Quoted in Joel Tena, "Death, Destruction, and Don't Forget the Strawberries," *California Aggie,* February 6, 1997.

are not based primarily on health considerations. . . . The current regulatory system does not, however, specifically consider infants and children. It does not examine the wide range of pesticide exposure patterns that appear to exist within the U.S. population.[28]

The NAS was confirming what many food-safety advocates had long contended: The pesticide tolerances set by the EPA were not strictly health-based standards. Instead, the EPA weighed the health risks against the pesticide's agricultural benefit and set tolerances that reflected the highest residue concentrations likely under normal use.[29]

HOW WE REGULATE PESTICIDES TODAY: THE FOOD QUALITY PROTECTION ACT

Throughout the period in which the NAS reports were being written and lawyers were engaged in attacking and defending the Delaney clause, Congress wasn't sitting on the sidelines. Every year, members of Congress filed bills and held hearings on pesticides and the Delaney clause. Though there was much discussion, there was no consensus on how to reform pesticide law to ensure safe use of pesticides. The agricultural community wanted the Delaney clause repealed, because they claimed that it barred too many safe uses of pesticides. The environmental and public health community would not agree to repeal the total ban on carcinogens in processed foods unless there would be a clear public health benefit.

Following the second NAS study, the benefits that pesticide reform offered became more apparent to health and environmental leaders. At that time, several key congressional staffers began to draft a compromise. The legislation they developed, the Food Quality Protection Act (FQPA), was a masterful piece of political craftsmanship. While it eliminated the Delaney clause's zero tolerance for cancer-causing pesticides that concentrate in processed foods, it also shifted the burden of proof from the government agencies to the pesticide manufacturers that a chemical was safe for the proposed use. If a company lacked sufficient evidence, the chemical would be subject to additional regulatory safeguards to protect human health. The bill also required the EPA to consider risks that it had ignored in the past, such as the impact of pesticides on children. These provisions help ensure that the EPA is equipped to take chemicals like Alar off the market much faster than before.

The FQPA passed both houses of Congress unanimously and was signed into law on August 3, 1996. In just a few weeks, Congress overturned 40 years of pesticide law. And surprisingly few people, especially in the agricultural or chemical industries, knew what powerful consumer safeguards the law would offer.

SAFER PESTICIDES AND SAFER FOOD: THE IMPACT OF THE FQPA

The Food Quality Protection Act provides three critical new protections for consumers. It requires the EPA to consider the special impact of pesticides on children when setting residue limits. It requires the agency to weigh the risks from multiple exposures to pesticides. Finally, it provides protections against pesticide effects other than cancer, such as disruption of the endocrine system. In the long run, this law will result in safer pesticides, safer food, and better information about which foods contain the most toxic pesticides. It was the most important food-safety law that Congress passed during the 1990s.

The new law gives the EPA 10 years to reassess the safety of all pesticides on the market, starting with the most hazardous ones first. The act also gives the EPA specific deadlines to inform Congress of its progress.

The first reporting deadline was August 1999, and it became clear then that the EPA had not completely followed the approach supported by Congress. According to an analysis of its actions by Consumers Union, instead of starting with the worst pesticides, the EPA largely stuck to the easiest pesticides, listing nearly 3,000 tolerances that were "obsolete or redundant." There was one notable exception. Right before the deadline passed, the EPA banned the use of a particularly toxic pesticide—methyl parathion—on food crops. Although the ban covered only 36 out of 113 uses of methyl parathion, it still represented a major food-safety improvement. The ban covered such foods as peaches, apples, pears, green beans, and grapes—foods especially popular with children. But it allowed the use of this pesticide on other food crops and cotton, where over 80 percent of the chemical was applied.[30] With the partial food ban on methyl parathion, the agency managed to reduce food-safety risks dramatically while minimizing the effect of the ban on most of the users.

Legal or approved pesticide residues are not the only problem. In a 1999 study, the Environmental Working Group, a nonprofit advocacy organization, found that the pesticide industry was taking advantage of a loophole in the new law to get emergency exemptions to use unapproved pesticides on fruits and vegetables commonly consumed by children. For example, since 1993, potatoes received 383 pesticide exemptions while tomatoes received 103. These exemptions clearly violate at least the spirit—if not the letter—of the FQPA, and should be stopped. The EPA should ensure that all pesticides in the diets of infants and children go though a rigorous review for their safety.[31]

Despite the EPA's slow start, continued implementation of the FQPA promises to deliver many future reductions in consumers' exposure to hazardous pesticides. However, this will occur only if many actors remain committed to implementating the law. The EPA has many tough pesticide issues to address under the act. Meanwhile, the pesticide industry and some farm groups are seeking to repeal sections of the act. Committed citizens and food-safety organizations need to remain vigilant to ensure that Congress doesn't backtrack and that the EPA fully enforces the law.

Protecting Children from Pesticides

Historically, tolerances for food have been set at levels considered safe for the average consumer, typically a man weighing between 140 and 160 pounds. But there can be a huge disparity between the levels of a toxic agent that are tolerated by that so-called average consumer and the levels that are safe for a pregnant woman or a developing child. The FQPA recognized that children are not simply young adults when it comes to setting pesticide tolerances. Children may eat particular foods in great quantities and, as any parent knows, can focus on a specific food or food group to the exclusion of all others. Children are also growing, which means that a toxic agent, consumed at a certain time, could have a particularly detrimental effect on their growth or development. Thus, children may be more susceptible than adults to harm from certain toxic pesticides.

The new pesticide law instructs the EPA, when reviewing a pesticide, to specifically consider its impact on children. The law requires the agency to analyze which foods children consume at a high frequency, children's special susceptibility, and the impact of cumulative effect from pesticide exposures.

Although this is one of the single most important sections of the law, its implementation is occurring at a snail's pace. And the food industry is finding loopholes, such as the emergency exemption requirement that has allowed farmers to continue to use unapproved and highly toxic pesticides on many fruits and vegetables.[32]

Evaluating Multiple Chemical Exposures

Prior to the FQPA, the EPA evaluated every pesticide use independently of every other one. While this approach may have been the easiest, it did not reflect real-world exposure to pesticide residues that occur from food, water, and environmental sources. The FQPA replaced the "zero cancer risk" standard that the Delaney clause established with a requirement that pesticide uses be safe. "Safe" is defined as providing consumers with "a reasonable certainty that no harm will result" from *all* exposures to a particular pesticide or similar pesticide.

This requirement represents a huge public health advance. However, it is another provision that the EPA has been slow to implement. Eventually, it may force the EPA and the pesticide industry to identify the most important uses for every pesticide, and then eliminate secondary ones, so that each pesticide can be retained for its most essential uses. In the long run, pesticide use may become more restricted, and this will create markets for alternative treatments to eliminate pests without the use of toxic chemicals.

Controlling Reproductive Effects of Pesticides

Some chemicals interact with the body in much the same way as the hormone estrogen does. These chemicals can have severe and potentially irreversible impacts, especially during growth and development of the fetus. These effects have already been documented in bird and fish species, where exposure to the insecticide DDT (dichlorodiphenyl-trichloroethane) and the industrial chemicals PCBs (polychlorinated biphenyls) has been linked to changes in the reproductive system of the offspring, sterility, and stunted growth.[33]

DDT, PCBs, and other chemicals suspected of causing those effects were banned in the 1970s. However, they persist in air, water, and soil. Residues of banned pesticides continue to be found in fish and many other foods, including baked goods, fruit, vegetables, meat, poultry, and dairy.

The risk posed by persistent chemicals with effects on the endocrine system were recognized during the development of the FQPA. The bill requires the industry and the EPA to consider whether a pesticide chemical mimics naturally occurring estrogen or has other endocrine effects.

The FQPA gave the EPA a new regulatory tool to reduce consumer exposure to chemicals likely to affect the human endocrine system: the use of an additional "tenfold" safety factor. The EPA may decrease the amount of pesticide allowed in food by a factor of 10 in order to reduce consumers' risk from the unknown effects of pesticide exposure. This additional safety factor provides a strong incentive for the chemical industry to conduct more rigorous testing of the potential health effects of each pesticide, in order to eliminate unknown health effects.

Although the FQPA will clearly benefit public health, the EPA still faces a daunting implementation task. The good news is that even though there are thousands of pesticide uses on food, the EPA could make foods much safer, especially for children, by banning or restricting the hundred riskiest pesticide uses.

"The simple fact is," says Ned Groth, senior scientific adviser at Consumers Union, "*most* uses of *most* pesticides on *most* foods do not leave residues that raise any public health concern. Out of nearly 10,000 registered food uses, only 100 or so uses—15 to 20 of the most hazardous pesticides, each used on a handful of foods—are responsible for the vast majority of dietary risk."

This means that the FQPA does not threaten the survival or profitability of agriculture, as some critics have alleged. But, by banning just a modest number of the most hazardous uses, it will result in better and safer use of pesticides on our food.

PICK CAREFULLY, WASH THOROUGHLY

Despite the real concerns about the possible effects of pesticides in your food, nearly two-thirds of the food analyzed by the FDA does not test positive for pesticide residues, and those that do are generally well below current government limits. And with implementation of the FQPA, things are only going to improve.

HOW TO REDUCE YOUR RISKS FROM PESTICIDES

1. Wash and peel fruits and vegetables.

2. Buy organic foods.

3. Buy conventionally grown foods with low pesticide residues.

4. Eat a variety of fruits and vegetables.

5. Seek up-to-date information on pesticide residues in food.

A number of sources are available to provide up-to-date information about which foods are most likely to contain pesticide residues. As we write this, *Consumer Reports* ranks only two foods as "very high concern" when it comes to pesticide residues: peaches grown in the United States and frozen winter squash. Other foods regularly eaten by children were found to be of "high concern," including apples, green beans grown in the United States, imported peaches, strawberries, and tomatoes grown in Mexico.[34] This analysis is likely to be updated in the future during the implementation period for the FQPA, and, over time, we expect to see fewer foods in the "very high" and "high" concern categories.

The advice on which foods are most likely to be contaminated is changing rapidly due to implementation of the new law. Therefore, seek guidance regularly from Consumers Union (publisher of *Consumer Reports*) and other groups.

Many consumer and environmental organizations have useful websites. For example, FoodNews.org, developed by the Environmental Working Group (EWG), allows you to visit a "virtual supermarket" and receive a report on the pesticide residues in what you purchased. On this website, EWG has collected all the government data available on different foods. As you "select items," the computer program randomly selects pesticide residue information on the same type of food as tested by the government. You can repeat the test several times to get a sense of your likely exposure. You can also use the site to obtain pesticide information on a virtual fruit salad or analyze your child's diet. We used this website and others to compile a list of conventionally grown foods that are likely to have few or no pesticide residues.

THE "VIRTUALLY" PESTICIDE-FREE SHOPPING CART

We took a trip into cyberspace to identify those food choices with the greatest likelihood of carrying no pesticide residues or only harmless ones. Using studies that analyze government food-testing data, we created this list of pesticide-safe foods grown conventionally. This doesn't necessarily mean that they were grown without using harmful pesticides, but that no (or very few) harmful pesticides remain in or on the foods when they reach the store. As the EPA further implements the Food Quality Protection Act, the list of foods you can buy without pesticide residues will likely grow.

Fruits	Vegetables	Cheeses
Bananas	Artichokes	Blue
Bitter melon	Asparagus	Camembert
Blueberries	Baked beans	Colby
Kiwi	Bamboo shoots	Edam
Mango	Beets (red)	Feta
Olives (stuffed)	Black-eyed peas	Gouda
Peaches (canned)	Brussels sprouts	Provolone
Pineapple (canned)	Cabbage	Reggiano
Watermelon	Cauliflower	Ricotta
	Corn	Romano
	Eggplant	
	Daikon	
	Garbanzo beans	
	Leeks	
	Lotus root	
	Okra	
	Onions	
	Peas	
	Pinto beans	
	Pumpkin	
	Radicchio	

Vegetables

Rhubarb
Shallots
Sweet corn (processed)
Sweet peas (processed)
Taro root
Tofu
Tomatillos
Water chestnuts

Other Dairy	Breads, Grains, Pastas	Meats
Cream	Basmati rice	Ham
Half-and-half	Cornflakes	Veal cutlet
Milk	Cracked wheat bread	
Yogurt	Glutinous rice	
Whipping cream	Jasmine rice	
	Sweet rice	

Seafood	Nuts	Other
Clams	Almonds	Apricot jelly
Flounder	Brazil nuts	Apple juice
Grouper	Cashews	Beer
Halibut	Chestnuts	Cherry jelly
Mahimahi	Coconuts	Chocolate syrup
Mussels	Peanuts	Coffee
Sardines	Pine nuts	French dressing
Scallops	Walnuts	Gelatin dessert
Tuna fillet		Grape juice
		Honey
		Italian dressing
		Maple syrup
		Olive oil
		Orange juice
		Peach juice
		Red raspberry jam

Other

Soy sauce
Strawberry jelly
Soybean oil
Tapioca

Sources: Environmental Working Group, www.foodnews.org; Consumers Union, www.ecologic-ipm.com/PDP/Table4_1998.pdf.

Choosing foods with little or no pesticide residues is getting easier and easier as organic products boasting a new national label arrive at your local market. After a decade of delay, the "USDA organic" label will finally make pesticide-free and pesticide-reduced foods more readily available. While there have been many organic labels and certifiers in the past, this has created confusion for consumers who can't always tell if one labeled product is better than another. The new organic label, which sets a nationwide standard for how organic food is grown, will clear up this confusion.

PESTICIDES ON THE PLATE?

To reduce your chances of being exposed to harmful pesticide residues, we suggest that you choose organic, especially for these fruits and vegetables:

Fruits	Vegetables
Apples	Celery
Cherries	Green beans
Grapes	Lettuce
Peaches	Spinach
Pears	Winter squash
Red raspberries	
Strawberries	

Consumers can reduce their levels of pesticide exposure dramatically by just replacing fruits and vegetables containing high levels of hazardous pesticides with organic items. For example, many parents can significantly reduce their children's pesticide exposure by switching to organically grown apples, peaches, and strawberries.

The final step to reducing your exposure to pesticides (as well as your risk of food poisoning) is to thoroughly wash and peel your fruits and vegetables. Washing means more than just passing a carrot under the faucet for a half a second. To most effectively remove pesticide residues, wash produce in a bowl of water that includes a drop or two of dish soap, then rinse the produce under cold running water. Washing doesn't eliminate all pesticide residues, but it certainly helps.

DRINKING WATER

Safe drinking water is a paramount health concern. While careful food choices can reduce the likelihood of microbial and chemical exposure, water is an essential element and an ingredient of many other foods. Americans who travel to developing countries are warned to avoid drinking the water, but at home we trust that the water from our tap is safe to drink. This is one luxury of living in a developed country that is not shared in many other countries. However, the safety of our drinking water is not something we can take for granted.

The Centers for Disease Control and Prevention (CDC) estimates that about 940,000 Americans get sick and 900 die each year from waterborne microbial illnesses caused by drinking water. Recent microbial outbreaks linked to water have demonstrated that more must be done to prevent harmful bacteria from contaminating the water supply. For example, in 1993 the largest waterborne-disease outbreak ever recorded in the United States happened in Milwaukee, Wisconsin. An estimated 403,000 people became ill, and 4,400 hospitalizations and 40 deaths resulted. The victims were infected by a parasite called *Cryptosporidium,* even though their drinking water had been filtered and chlorinated.[35]

Chemicals pose additional concerns. Many of the pesticides applied to farms can contaminate either groundwater or lakes and streams that are sources of drinking water, increasing the chance for consumer exposure to pesticide residues. The leaching of pesticide chemicals from farms, homes, and commercial areas into water is called non-point source pollution. Unfortunately, this type of pollution is not controlled under the Clean Water Act.

Groundwater is a source of drinking water for approximately 46 percent of the U.S. population, including nearly everyone who lives in rural areas. It supplies 40 percent of the water in public water systems. In 1998, a survey of 26 states reported that in the aquifers tested, pesticides contaminated 31 percent and nitrates were found in 22 percent.[36]

Agricultural chemicals also often contaminate lakes and rivers. Pesticides are carried by runoff into surface waters, and their concentrations in surface water frequently correlate with pesticide applications in the planting season. Surface water, which includes all rivers, streams, lakes, and estuaries, contributes about 60 percent of the water in public water systems and supplies drinking water to the population that doesn't use groundwater. A recent study of a widely used pesticide, atrazine, indicates that some pesticides are contaminating the groundwater first and then flowing into the surface water, which further complicates the problem.[37]

Pesticides aren't the only problem. One deadly *E. coli* outbreak in Ontario, Canada, occurred after manure got into the wells used for drinking water, killing 7 and sickening 2,300. And an estimated 50 to 70 percent of the nutrients reaching surface waters, mainly nitrogen and phosphorus, come from fertilizers and animal waste on agricultural land. Nitrate, a very mobile ion containing nitrogen, is increasing in the nation's water supply, especially in the mid-continent. Infants under six months of age are most vulnerable to exposure to nitrates, as it may lead to the fatal "blue baby syndrome."[38]

The EPA sets standards for the safety of drinking water. Starting in 1974, the Safe Drinking Water Act adopted two dozen standards as mandatory requirements. These standards, developed by the U.S. Public Health Service, had previously been adopted by some local water authorities on a voluntary basis and were quite weak. One standard was for arsenic in drinking water, which was developed in 1942 based on very limited science.

BOTTLED WATER

While many consumers think that bottled water is safer than tap water, it is subject to weak and crisis-driven oversight from the FDA. In fact, government and industry surveys have found that an estimated 25 percent of bottled waters were merely packaged tap water. Sometimes bottled tap water is treated further; sometimes it is not. And when the Natural Resources Defense Council surveyed over a thousand bottles of water, it found that about one-third of the 103 brands tested violated enforceable state standards or microbial or chemical guidelines, or both. In fact, more regulatory standards are in place for tap water than for bottled water in both the United States and Europe, even though bottled water sells for up to 1,000 times the price of tap water. *

* Ibid., Executive Summary; World Wildlife Fund, "The Real Cost of Bottled Water," news release, May 3, 2001.

The Arsenic Connection

Arsenic—a well-known poison—is widely distributed throughout the earth's crust. It usually enters the water supply through erosion, fossil-fuel combustion, and commercial applications. The intake of arsenic through drinking water and other sources has been linked to an increased cancer risk in many organs, including skin, lungs, bladder, and kidney.[39]

The Safe Drinking Water Act has been amended several times, most recently in 1996. The 1996 amendments adopted many changes also made in the Food Quality Protection Act. For example, Congress directed the EPA to consider the risk to vulnerable consumers, including children, when setting safety standards for drinking water. The EPA can also require that drinking water be screened for the presence of estrogenic chemicals and other endocrine disrupters.

The 1996 amendments required the EPA to set a new standard for arsenic in drinking water, since the old one had been set in the 1940s before scientists knew that arsenic could cause cancer. Over the decades, many expert scientific and public health bodies have recommended that the standard for arsenic be reevaluated. In 1999, the National Academy of Sciences issued a report concluding that the arsenic standard "does not

---

The 1996 amendments to the Safe Drinking Water Act required the government for the first time to set standards for bottled water. The new standards, when they are set, should be at least equivalent to those governing tap water. These new protections should address gaps and gaffes, like the benzene that contaminated Perrier, a well-known bottled water imported from France. * The law also directs water providers to inform their customers about the safety of the drinking water at least annually. New York and Massachusetts are among the few states that maintain lists of bottled water sources. To learn the sources of bottled water, call those state programs or the bottler.

* Erik Olson et al., *Bottled Water: Pure Drink or Pure Hype?* (New York: Natural Resources Defense Council, 1999), chap. 4, available at www.nrdc.org.

achieve EPA's goal for public health protection and therefore requires downward revision as promptly as possible."[40]

In January 2001, as the Clinton administration prepared to leave Washington, the EPA finalized its revised standard for arsenic, reducing it from 50 parts per billion (ppb) to 10 ppb, the same standard adopted by the World Health Organization and the European Union.[41] Shortly after Bush took office, his administration suspended the arsenic-in-drinking-water standard. This decision was an early hallmark of the Bush administration's attitudes toward environmental issues. Then, in October 2001, in the wake of additional scientific study, the administration reversed course and adopted the Clinton administration's approach.

Learning About Your Water's Safety

Thanks to the 1996 amendments to the Safe Drinking Water Act, more information on contaminants in drinking water is available than ever before. Congress directed large local water providers to mail annual reports to their customers with information on (1) the levels of regulated contaminants detected in tap water; (2) what the legal limits and the health goals are for those contaminants; (3) the levels of some unregulated contaminants found in the water; (4) the system's compliance with health standards and other requirements; (5) the health effects of regulated contaminants found in drinking water; and (6) an EPA hot line where you can get more information. While smaller water authorities don't have to mail these reports, you can still get a copy if you call your local provider (to which you pay your water bill).[42]

Call your water provider to get information on the levels of arsenic and other contaminants in your tap water, then compare it with the EPA's list of Current Drinking Water Standards (available at www.epa.gov/safewater/mcl.html). If your water provider won't provide it, write a letter to the editor of your local newspaper. You have a right to know what risks may exist in your tap water. By learning about any contaminants, you can make a more informed decision about whether to choose bottled or tap water.

OTHER CHEMICALS/OTHER CONCERNS

Pesticides are just one group of chemicals that may contaminate our food. Numerous industrial and environmental chemicals show up in a broad range of foods, from fish to milk. Some persist in the environment for long periods and can enter the food supply through a variety of channels. Cattle might graze on grass that contains minute particles of airborne dioxin. Shellfish and lobsters live in shallow coastal areas that may be polluted with PCBs. Sharks and other predatory fish may accumulate methylmercury and toxins from the other fish that make up their diet. Through a process called bioaccumulation, fish and animals at the top of the food chain—like sharks, swordfish, and humans—accumulate higher levels of environmental chemicals in their bodies. Over time, these fish and animals accumulate chemical residues in their fat at levels much higher than any of their contributing food sources. The effects of these chemicals on humans may be serious and insidious—although difficult to measure.

After 50 years of emphasis on the cancer-causing potential of contaminants in food, health experts are now increasingly studying other health hazards. One study done by Sandra and Joseph Jacobson indicates that the effects of some chemicals in our diet may be multigenerational. Those effects include learning disabilities and lower IQs in children born to mothers with high chemical exposure levels.[43] *Our Stolen Future,* a landmark book by scientist Theo Colborn and others, describes how certain chemicals in the diet, called endocrine disrupters, may be having very serious effects on the reproductive systems of humans. These effects, like reduced sperm counts in men and endometriosis in women, were never contemplated or controlled by environmental and food-safety laws until passage of the Food Quality Protection Act. While many of these risks are largely theoretical, they deserve careful study.

Mercury

Mercury is a persistent environmental chemical that causes adverse health effects at lower doses than would be required to cause cancer. This heavy metal is found naturally on Earth and in the atmosphere. Inorganic mercury enters the atmosphere from coal and industrial emissions, then falls to the earth and enters the water supply. Bacteria combine mercury and carbon to form methylmercury. This form of mercury contaminates fish muscle as fish feed in contaminated waters. When a predator fish, like a shark, eats many small contaminated fish over the course of its life, the methylmercury concentrates. Human consumption compounds the accumulation further.

The "mad hatters" of Lewis Carroll's time were adult victims of mercury poisoning, since they absorbed some of the mercury used in the production of felt hats. Depression and loss of memory were among their early symptoms. With larger doses of mercury, the victims became psychotic, suffered hallucinations and delusions, and became demented, like the Mad Hatter in *Alice's Adventures in Wonderland*.[44]

In another well-known mercury-poisoning episode, an entire Japanese town suffered from pollution of its local waterways. Minamata, a small factory town facing the Shiranui Sea, was dominated by a petrochemical and plastic-making company that released mercury into the harbor. People living around the harbor experienced numbness in limbs and lips, slurred speech, constricted vision, serious brain damage, unconsciousness, or involuntary shaking. When the company started dumping wastes into the Minamata River, the same "illness" developed in the people living around the river. The Minamata episode also helped to establish the connection between mercury poisoning and fetal effects.[45]

In 1991 and again in 2000, the National Academy of Sciences concluded that children of symptom-free pregnant and nursing mothers with relatively low levels of mercury as measured in their hair and blood may suffer adverse health effects from prenatal mercury exposure. These symptoms include delayed motor activity, delayed speech, cerebral palsy, and mental retardation.[46] These conclusions were based on a review of the relationship of clinical signs in humans to blood, hair, and urine mercury levels in a number of human poisoning episodes, including Minamata, and in studies of fish-eating populations.

Today, Americans are exposed to methylmercury when we eat contaminated fish, but the mercury is not in doses large enough to cause obvious poisoning. However, FDA safety standards for commercial seafood were developed without considering methylmercury's effects on children exposed in utero. This means that pregnant women who eat a lot of swordfish, shark, tuna, and other fish with high mercury levels may be unintentionally harming their unborn children.

Consuming fish caught from lakes and rivers polluted with mercury can also harm unborn children. Many states have warned pregnant women and children to avoid fish from local waterways.[47] However, warnings vary by state, and this has led to consumer confusion. Many public health groups and scientists believe that the federal government should set strong national public health standards and issue clear advice about fish consumption.

The FDA's failure to issue credible government warnings about methylmercury in fish has already had irreversible public health consequences. The CDC, in a national survey of exposure patterns among women and children, found nearly 1 in 10 women had mercury levels very close to toxic levels. These findings place a significant number of women and children each year at risk of adverse effects from mercury in their diet.[48]

Women who are or may become pregnant should avoid or limit top-of-the-food-chain fish such as shark, swordfish, king mackerel, tuna (steaks), or white or golden snapper. While canned tuna is safer than tuna steaks, women who are (or trying to become) pregnant should limit their intake of canned tuna to 5 ounces a week (or one drained 6-ounce can). Children under 25 pounds should have no more than 2.5 ounces of canned tuna a month, or about half a can (one homemade sandwich). From 25 to 45 pounds, they can eat another sandwich (2.5 ounces) each month. For every 15 pounds after that, the maximum amount per month increases by one homemade tuna fish sandwich until they reach the recommended adult maximum of 7 ounces (three sandwiches) per week.[49]

Dioxins and PCBs

Dioxins, furans, and PCBs are related chemicals that are suspected endocrine disrupters, which means they can mimic or interfere with the effects of hormones. Dioxins are also potent carcinogens—in fact, one type, TCDD, has the dubious distinction of being the most potent animal carcinogen ever tested.

PCBs are a class of industrial chemicals that are highly stable, heat-resistant, and nonflammable. PCBs have been used widely in electrical transformer fluids, hydraulic fluids, and heat transfer fluids, as well as lubricants, coatings, and inks. The Toxic Substances Control Act of 1974 outlawed the manufacture and import of PCBs. But, like asbestos, they remain a continuing hazard in our surroundings, such as in the electrical transformers in old buildings. The FDA calls PCBs "a persistent and ubiquitous contaminant," because they don't break down naturally.[50]

PCBs and dioxins contaminate the food chain as a result of pollution. They spill into water during industrial accidents or from old dumpsites, and they go up in smoke when, for example, a hot fire destroys an old building. In fact, municipal and hospital waste incinerators are major sources of dioxin emissions, although these are being reduced thanks to improved government controls.

Fish, wildlife, and livestock ingest PCBs and dioxins as they eat. Freshwater fish and seafood can carry the highest levels of dioxins and PCBs. In fact, 29 percent of all fish advisories are caused by PCBs, and 82 percent of those occur in the states that border the Great Lakes.[51]

PCBs and dioxins have been linked to numerous adverse effects in both humans and wildlife, including a number of acute episodes. These types of exposures are rare, but clearly excess exposure to this family of chemicals should be avoided.

- A 1976 explosion in a chemical plant in Seveso, Italy, spread airborne dioxins over a large geographic region and the rate of male births in the area declined.[52]

- The dioxins in Agent Orange, a herbicide, are the suspected cause of cases of spina bifida among children of Vietnam veterans, as well as being associated with soft-tissue sarcoma, Hodgkin's disease, and non-Hodgkin's lymphoma. They have also recently been linked to type II diabetes.[53]

- PCB intake has been correlated to developmental delays and lower IQ scores in the children of women who ate large quantities of tainted fish from the Great Lakes during pregnancy. Recent studies document that PCBs can also adversely affect adult learning and memory.[54]

The good news is that effective environmental pollution controls have reduced our exposure to dioxin and PCBs over the last 20 years.

Even so, a 2000 EPA Draft Dioxin Reassessment estimated that people who eat large quantities of high-fat foods (which contain the most dioxin) face a risk of cancer as high as 1 in 100. Over 90 percent of our exposure comes from animal products: fish, beef, poultry, and non-skim dairy. You can cut a lot of dioxin out of your diet just by reducing meat consumption and cutting the fat. This is great nutritional advice as well. If you do eat meat, choose leaner cuts of meat, like sirloin, round steak, or pork tenderloin. Eat chicken breast or drumstick instead of the fattier thigh. Trim the skin off both poultry and fish to reduce dioxin exposure. Choosing lower-fat dairy items will also help.[55]

Marine fish that spent most of their life in deep oceans will be less likely to carry dioxins and PCBs than the freshwater varieties. But some marine fish, like rockfish, striped bass, snapper, and redfish, may also contain dioxin because they spend part of their lives breeding close to shore. Lower-fat seafood will carry less of the harmful chemicals, but don't eat the green tomalley in lobster, which can carry a big dose.[56]

Chemical concerns should not dissuade women from breast-feeding their infants. Although breast milk can contain environmental chemicals, experts say that the benefits still outweigh the risks. [57]

CHAPTER FIVE

TEN STEPS TO A HEALTHY DIET

In the 1970s movie classic *Sleeper*, health-food-store owner Woody Allen wakes up 200 years in the future in a society where doctors and scientists have turned conventional food wisdom upside down. Foods like steak, hot fudge, and cream pies are now considered the keys to good health. Moviegoers found this especially funny because it played on the common impression that the medical community is constantly changing its mind about what we should eat. News stories seem regularly to announce unexpected, startling research results, such as the finding that small amounts of alcohol taken daily lower the risk of heart disease.

But even as scientists refine their understanding of nutrition and occasionally reach unanticipated conclusions that overturn food orthodoxy, the basics of good nutrition have remained quite constant over the past several decades. If we ignore the food fads and overpublicized news reports of preliminary studies of relatively few people, nutrition advice looks much less fickle. To reduce the risk of disease, avoid weight gain, and feel healthy, the safest and surest course is to follow the well-established principles of good nutrition.

Most people know these principles—for example, avoid overeating; eat plenty of fruits and vegetables; limit consumption of salt, sugar, and fats—but it can be hard to put them into practice. For one thing, many of the things that should be avoided, such as chocolate candy bars, soft drinks, french fries, and hamburgers, taste good and are fun to eat.

Of course, none of those foods is lethal or needs to be entirely avoided, but it can be maddeningly difficult to keep their consumption in check and eat enough of more nutritious foods. For example, when the U.S. Department of Agriculture (USDA) conducted a national survey of nutritional knowledge and eating behavior, 68 percent of adults stated that it was "very important" to them to "choose a diet with plenty of fruits and vegetables," yet only 23 percent of Americans ate as much fruit as recommended by the USDA's Dietary Guidelines and only 22 percent of Americans ate as much as they themselves perceived to be necessary for good health. Similarly, many of the 58 percent of Americans who said it was very important to eat a diet low in fat nevertheless thought they ate too much fat, and indeed most of them consumed more than recommended in the Dietary Guidelines.[1]

As increasing numbers of people eat meals on the run or in restaurants where unhealthy food choices far outnumber the good ones, the temptation to eat a high-fat, high-cholesterol, high-salt, high-sugar, disease-causing diet can be overwhelming. When Americans eat at home, they get 32 percent of their calories from fat, only a little more than the 30 percent maximum recommended in the Dietary Guidelines; but when they eat out, fat comprises 38 percent of their calories.[2]

To make matters worse, the industries that produce the foods that are worst for us—including snacks, fast foods, soft drinks, and meat—bombard us with ads. Between mediocre diets and sedentary lifestyles, it's no wonder that a growing number of people are overweight or otherwise at risk from heart disease, diabetes, and other diseases that have at least part of their root causes in poor nutrition. Not only has the percentage of adults who are overweight increased, but one out of seven schoolchildren is obese—twice as many as 20 years ago.[3]

Yale University diet expert Kelly Brownell observes, "Our diet is deteriorating and physical activity is declining." Good public policies could help improve matters—nutrition campaigns in the media, restrictions on the sale of junk food in school cafeterias, more funding for public recreation facilities—but, in the meantime, we need to focus on individual efforts to provide ourselves and our families with a healthy diet.[4]

A study by the U.S. Department of Health and Human Services concluded that at least 300,000 deaths a year are caused by poor diet and lack of physical activity. For one thing, scientists have proven conclusively that diet plays an important role in heart disease. Too much saturated and *trans* fat and cholesterol—derived largely from meat, dairy products, pastries, and eggs—raise cholesterol. Insufficient fiber, folate, and possibly omega-3 fats (like the fat in fish) leave the heart unprotected. In one study, men with high cholesterol were able to improve their blood flow by cutting down on fat and eating more fruits, vegetables, nuts, and whole grains.[5]

Diet also plays a key role in cutting the risk of other diseases. You can lower your risk of high blood pressure and stroke by avoiding excess weight, excess alcohol, too much sodium, and too little potassium. A diet that's low in saturated fat and rich in fruits and vegetables and low-fat dairy products can also keep blood pressure low. Staying lean, eating plenty of fruits and vegetables, and cutting back on red meat may also cut the risk of some cancers.

You can drastically cut your risk of diabetes by staying lean. Excess weight is by far the leading cause of diabetes, responsible for more than 80 percent of the adult cases. On the positive side, getting enough calcium and vitamin D keeps bones strong and lower the risk of osteoporosis.[6]

This chapter offers 10 steps to a healthy diet. It will give you suggestions for how to put sound nutrition principles into practice and avoid the ever-present bad food temptations out there. Unlike the advice in some diet books, these steps will provide you with a way of eating that can last a lifetime. They will help you make relatively simple and gradual changes that add up to major improvements.

If, in addition to maximizing your general health and avoiding heart disease, you want to reduce your weight, these same diet suggestions are appropriate. They will help you reduce the number of calories you consume, and that remains the undisputable key to weight loss, along with exercise. Doctors, nutritionists, and scientists have conducted numerous studies that show that if you cut any type of calories from your diet—whether it be protein, fat, sugar, or carbohydrates—you will lose weight. Some people may find it easier to reduce their total caloric intake by eating a high-protein diet, while others may prefer to focus on foods with few calories for their weight (such as vegetables, fruits, and low-fat dairy and poultry), but it is still the number of calories that ultimately counts. A short-term specialized diet may help you lose excess pounds, but you should return quickly to a healthful diet grounded in the principles of good nutrition.

TEN STEPS TO A HEALTHY DIET

1. Don't supersize your portions.
2. Eat less margarine, butter, and shortening.
3. Cut down on egg yolks.
4. Choose nonfat and low-fat dairy.
5. Select whole grains.
6. Eat less meat.
7. Fill up on vegetables.
8. Cut the salt.
9. Make fruits your snacks.
10. Avoid sugar.

1. DON'T SUPERSIZE YOUR PORTIONS

Over the past several decades, Americans have eaten larger and larger servings, thereby increasing their caloric intake. What was once a feast is now an average meal.

Restaurants have helped stimulate this trend. "In the 1950s and 1960s," report Bonnie Liebman and David Schardt in the *Nutrition Action Healthletter,*

> McDonald's offered only one size of french fries. It weighed over two ounces and contained roughly 200 calories, like today's "small." In the early 1970s, the original fries became a small, and a 320-calorie large size was introduced. In the 1980s, the 1970s large became a medium and the new large swelled to 400 calories. By the mid 90s, the large had grown to 450 calories and customers could now order a "super size" with 540 calories. By 2000, the large had become medium, the super size had become large, and the new seven-ounce super size had ballooned to 610 calories.[7]

People who buy a supersize McDonald's value meal, consisting of a quarter-pound hamburger with cheese, fries, and a Coke, take in more than 1,500 calories—three-quarters of an adult's average daily needs. Because the additional cost to McDonald's for larger portions is small, the company increases profits by encouraging consumers to buy ever-larger sizes and strengthens customer loyalty by seeming to offer a good deal.

Other fast-food chains have gotten on the supersize bandwagon. Jack in the Box has periodically offered a Triple Ultimate Cheeseburger, for example. This one sandwich provides more than half of a day's recommended calories and even more than a day's fat intake (84 grams versus the recommended 65 grams). The Burger King Double Whopper with Cheese is nearly as bad.[8]

Sit-down restaurants similarly try to convince customers that they are getting their money's worth by providing so much food that they leave feeling stuffed. Steakhouses like Outback offer a 20-ounce porterhouse steak with about 1,150 calories. A full meal with dessert can easily exceed twice that amount. A seemingly more modest meal such as the mushroom cheeseburger, fries, and Coke at Applebee's tilts the scale at 1,700 calories. An appetizer of chicken wings or fried mozzarella sticks or a fudge brownie sundae can add more than 1,000 additional calories.[9]

Because Americans are eating an increasing number of meals in restaurants, these feast-sized portions are becoming an everyday occurrence. And those restaurant-sized serving portions can be even more damaging if we begin eating similar amounts at home.

Snack packages and individual desserts have also been creeping up in size. Candy bars used to be about 1.5 ounces, but now many stores feature king-size bars of two, three, or more ounces. A medium-sized movie theater serving of popcorn with butter can provide more than 1,000 calories. In one almost unbelievable example, the Cheesecake Factory offers a slice of carrot cake with 1,560 calories and 83 grams of fat.[10]

To deal with serving-size inflation, consciously keep the portions down when you're eating at home. The serving sizes on the Nutrition Facts labels on foods are a good guide to an appropriate amount for most items. Decide how much you are going to eat before sitting down at the table, and then don't go back for seconds.

When eating out, try to avoid restaurants that only serve humongous quantities and resist the temptations of all-you-can-eat buffets. You can split an entrée with a friend or plan in advance to eat only half of what you're served and take the rest home to eat later. Many of us grew up being told to finish everything on our plate, because "there are children starving in China," but we need to resist eating every morsel that's served, since it's our health and waistlines that will suffer.

2. EAT LESS MARGARINE, BUTTER, AND SHORTENING

The butter and margarine we add to our food is a big waste of calories and sometimes promotes heart disease. Find healthier, equally delicious ways to flavor your food. This is one easy way to improve your diet and help your waistline.

Butter is loaded with artery-clogging saturated fat. Ordinary stick-type margarine contains hydrogenated oils that make it about as bad for your heart as butter. Instead, choose a lower-fat or nonfat tub margarine.

Luckily, there are lots of alternatives. For toast, try honey, jam, fruit spreads, or a "butter" spray. For steamed zucchini and other hot vegetables, lemon juice and a dash of oregano add some zip. Try nutmeg on cooked carrots and garlic and a touch of olive oil on spinach. For baked potatoes, fat-free sour cream or salsa is delicious. If you simply can't give up butter, buy a whipped light butter or use just a little of the real thing.

Many packaged and restaurant foods contain partially hydrogenated oils and shortening that clog arteries. Cut way back on french fries, fried chicken, fried fish, doughnuts, cakes, and similar foods. For your sweet tooth, choose low-fat or fat-free cookies or cakes.

Even ordinary vegetable oil can be a problem because of its calories. In fact, the oil in salad dressing is the biggest source of fat for many people. Even the best oils, olive and canola, have as many calories as butter or soybean oil, even though they are low in saturated fat and friendly to your heart. For sautéing, use water or broth, a vegetable-oil spray, or a small amount of olive or canola oil. Choose fat-free or low-fat salad dressings. When you are cooking, use less oil or shortening than the recipes call for.

Thousands of packaged foods offer unnecessary fat. Look for baked foods that are just about as tasty, but much lower in fat and calories. Buy baked potato or tortilla chips, low-fat cookies and cakes, baked ramen noodle soup, and low-fat frozen french fries instead of the traditional versions.

In your effort to cut down on fat, avoid turning to the synthetic fat olestra, sold under the brand name Olean. It can cause diarrhea, abdominal cramps, flatulence, and other adverse effects, which can sometimes be severe. Even more important, it reduces your body's ability to absorb fat-soluble carotenoids, such as lycopene and lutein, from fruits and vegetables. Many experts believe these nutrients lower the risk of cancer, heart disease, and other health problems.

3. CUT DOWN ON EGG YOLKS

Eggs are versatile, convenient, and tasty. Too bad one egg yolk contains almost a day's worth of cholesterol. That cholesterol clogs arteries, promoting heart disease and stroke. The fewer egg yolks—and the less cholesterol—you consume, the better.

When cooking, think of yolks in eggs like you would the bones in chicken—and just discard them instead of eating them. It's easy to make tasty scrambled egg dishes with just egg whites or egg substitutes like Egg Beaters.

For many recipes, such as pancakes and waffles, you can replace one whole egg with two whites. When you're preparing a recipe that calls for two whole eggs, experiment with one whole egg and two whites; the next time with four whites.

At fast-food restaurants, avoid egg-containing sandwiches and muffins. At regular restaurants, look for egg-white omelettes on the menu or ask the chef to prepare eggs with egg whites or an egg substitute.

4. CHOOSE NONFAT OR LOW-FAT DAIRY

Whole milk, cheese, and ice cream are tasty and rich in calcium. But they are also loaded with saturated fat and cholesterol, which promote heart disease. Therefore, look for ways to change your dairy food habit.

Switching to skim or 1 percent milk is one of the most important changes that most people could make. Over a lifetime, the average one-glass-a-day milk drinker, by drinking skim instead of whole milk (3.5 percent milkfat), would consume 400 pounds less fat—*that's 1.6 million calories!* If you have difficulty getting used to the taste of fat-free milk, you can buy nonfat milk that is produced using a process that gives it the richer taste of 2 percent milk.

The dairy industry now produces low-fat or fat-free versions of everything from milk to cream cheese to frozen yogurt. Those foods have all (or more) of the calcium and other nutrients that occur in old-fashioned, high-fat dairy products.

If you like ice cream, try sorbet, fat-free frozen yogurt, and fat-free ice cream. But don't go overboard—they are still loaded with sugar and calories.

By contrast, fat-free cheeses are too often taste-free as well. But most supermarkets have a dizzying array of reduced-fat cheeses that taste great. Over a few months, try the various lower-fat cheeses in your neighborhood grocery and keep track of which ones you like. If you can't give up regular cheese, at least have a smaller portion—make a cheese sandwich with one slice instead of two.

At restaurants, skip some or all of the cheese on sandwiches and in salads. Ask for half—or none—of the cheese on a pizza topped with tomato sauce and lots of vegetables.

5. SELECT WHOLE GRAINS

Start enjoying whole grain varieties of breads, cereals, and other foods. They'll add loads of flavor and variety to your meals—and provide more vitamins, minerals, and fiber than white bread, white rice, and other "re-fined" grains.

Fiber, the indigestible part of whole grains, has long been known to prevent constipation. It may also reduce the risk of diverticulosis and heart disease. Most of the fiber is lost when whole wheat flour or brown rice is milled and refined.

You can buy ordinary whole wheat bread (make sure that whole wheat is the only wheat-flour ingredient) in a supermarket, or find a far more delicious, crusty whole grain bread at a local bakery, or bake a loaf yourself. Eat it plain, or top it with apple butter, honey, low-fat tub margarine, low-fat cream cheese, or a few brushstrokes of olive oil.

One great thing about whole grains (and vegetables, beans, and other fiber-rich foods) is that they tend to be filling, and that helps control calories. If you load up on whole grains (and fruits and vegetables), you will almost certainly eat fewer foods high in fat and sugar.

To switch to a whole grain diet, you can start with the items on this shopping list:

- Whole grain cereals like Shredded Wheat, Wheaties, Cheerios, Raisin Bran, Kashi, All-Bran, 100 percent bran, oatmeal, or Wheatena

- A loaf of whole wheat sandwich bread

- A loaf of crusty whole wheat bread from a bakery

- A package of whole wheat pita bread

- Whole wheat pasta and whole wheat couscous (*superfast* to cook) from a health-food store

- Long-grain brown rice (try basmati for extra flavor) and a box of quick-cooking brown rice

- A package of whole wheat tortillas for making wraps with beans, rice, and diced sautéed vegetables

6. EAT LESS MEAT

For many people, eating less meat is the toughest dietary change to make—but the most important. Red meat is a major source of saturated fat and cholesterol, which are major causes of heart disease. Meat has also been linked to cancer of the colon and the prostate.

Even modest servings are loaded with saturated fat. A 4-ounce hamburger or 12-ounce sirloin steak (the leanest meat at a steak house) can use up nearly half a day's worth of saturated fat.

A "perfect diet" needn't eliminate *all* meat, but you should only eat small or occasional portions of the leanest meat (round or sirloin steak; pork tenderloin) and trim them carefully.

Chicken and turkey are lower in saturated fat than red meat. But it's still important to choose lower-fat varieties, such as the breast (second best: drumstick). Thighs and wings are fattier. In any case, always remove the skin. Figure 8 lists some of your meat choices, ranging from the best to the worst in saturated fat, before rounding. The numbers in the chart are for four ounces cooked.[11] Keep in mind that high-fat preparation methods, such as frying chicken or marinating steak in oil, can make these numbers much worse.

To get in the habit of consuming less meat, try not eating *any* meat or poultry for a week. As we saw in chapter 3, this will also be good for the environment.

FIGURE 8
MEAT: CALORIES AND FAT CONTENT
(4-ounce serving)

	Calories	Saturated fat (grams)	Total fat (grams)
Turkey breast (skinless)	153	0	1
Chicken breast (skinless)	186	1	4
Turkey leg (skinless)	180	1	4
Beef eye of round (select grade, carefully trimmed)	182	2	5
Chicken drumstick (skinless)	194	2	6
Beef top round (select, carefully trimmed)	226	2	6
Pork tenderloin (carefully trimmed)	211	3	7
Chicken breast (with skin)	223	3	9
Beef tip round (select, carefully trimmed)	210	3	8
Pork center loin (carefully trimmed)	228	3	9
Chicken drumstick (with skin)	244	3	13
Beef top round (choice grade, untrimmed)	253	5	12
Chicken wing (with skin)	328	6	22
Pork loin center rib (untrimmed, boneless)	294	7	18
Ground beef, 17% fat	289	7	19
Beef top sirloin (choice, untrimmed)	304	8	19
Ground beef, 27% fat	327	9	23
Porterhouse steak (choice, untrimmed)	345	10	25
Beef chuck blade roast (choice)	393	12	29
Pork spareribs (untrimmed)	449	13	34
Beef short ribs (choice, untrimmed)	532	20	47

Eschewing meat may sound less tempting than chewing it, but what *is* tempting is the enormous variety of delicious meatless dishes:

- Pizza topped with loads of vegetables (and half the cheese)
- Pasta topped with tomato sauce and steamed zucchini or broccoli
- Frozen veggie burgers (such as Gardenburgers or Boca Burgers) with vegetable side dishes
- A hearty homemade or canned lentil soup with crusty whole wheat bread.

As you cut down on meat, you should make beans a regular part of your diet. They are nutritional powerhouses, with lots of fiber and minerals. Many of them also have considerable protein, substituting for the protein you had been getting from meat and poultry. A cup of cooked lentils, one of the best beans, includes 25 percent of daily requirements for protein plus 57 percent of daily requirements for fiber, 19 percent for

THE EDIBLE SCHOOLYARD

Influential chef Alice Waters has said that the most neglected room in most schools is the lunchroom. If the purpose of schooling is to prepare young people for healthy, productive, fulfilling lives, then America's schools have been failing when it comes to food. As Waters notes, "In many schools, a bank of vending machines is the main attraction, and kids fill up on Cokes and snack foods. If there is a cafeteria, what it offers usually fails to meet the minimum guidelines for nutrition developed by the U.S. Department of Agriculture." Kids learn to prefer food that's bad for their health and bad for the environment.

At the inner-city Martin Luther King Jr. Middle School in Waters's hometown of Berkeley, California, there wasn't even a cafeteria. Instead, students lined up to buy packaged pizza from a concession stand or grabbed candy from the corner store. Waters, whose restaurant, Chez Panisse, pioneered the move toward cuisine based on fresh, local, organic ingredients, decided to approach the school.

Working with the school's principal, teachers, and community members, she planned an "edible schoolyard" and raised the money for it. In the spring of 1997, a two-acre garden replaced what had been an asphalt parking lot. With a gardening teacher, the students chose what

potassium, 81 percent for folic acid, 16 percent for magnesium, 33 percent for iron, 23 percent for copper, 15 percent for zinc, and 16 percent for vitamin B_6.[12] That's an impressive tally!

7. FILL UP ON VEGETABLES

Vegetables are key to a healthy diet. They contain relatively few calories and are brimming with vitamins, minerals, fiber, and phytochemicals that may protect against cancer, heart disease, stroke, and other maladies. Numerous studies have shown the many health benefits. For example, a recent analysis of the health records of 15,000 male doctors found that those men who daily ate at least two and a half servings of carotenoid-rich vegetables, such as broccoli, carrots, and spinach, reduced their risk of heart disease by 23 percent compared with those who ate less than one serving a day.[13]

---

to grow. They learned organic gardening techniques and began to produce everything from broccoli and bok choy to basil, blackberries, and bush beans.

But Waters wanted the students to learn more than just how to plant, weed, and harvest. She wanted to "seduce them into a whole new way of thinking about food" and to understand the interrelationship among food, land, and community. She worked with the school to establish a kitchen classroom where the students could prepare, eat, and discuss what they had grown. Teachers now link the garden and the kitchen to the curricula in science, history, and other subjects.

While the typical school teaches students to eat hamburgers, Twinkies, and potato chips, the Edible Schoolyard encourages its student gardeners to value the wide range of fresh, unprocessed whole foods. As one student remarked, "I didn't know what arugula was, but now I do, and I get my mom to go to the farmers' market and we have it in our salad."

Other schools in California, Ohio, and elsewhere have been adopting the Edible Schoolyard model. To learn how to start an interdisciplinary school-garden project, you can get a 92-page guide titled *The Edible Schoolyard*, available through the Center for Ecoliteracy at www.ecoliteracy.org.

The National Cancer Institute recommends eating at least five to nine half-cup servings a day of vegetables and fruit. Eat them raw, steamed, or sautéed. Eat them as main courses, snacks, or side dishes. When you eat lots of vegetables, you'll have much less room in your stomach for fatty foods—so you might lose a few pounds without even trying.

Following the National Cancer Institute's slogan of "5 a Day" is easiest when you make vegetables the main course, such as sautéed vegetables on rice or a thick lentil-vegetable soup with whole wheat bread and salad. That way you're sure to get several servings' worth in one meal. You might experiment with a vegetarian diet, even if it's only a couple of days a week.

Some vegetables are better for you than others since they include more vitamins, minerals, and fiber. Be sure to include some of those in your diet. The chart below lists the top 10 vegetables from a nutrition standpoint, along with those at the bottom of the list (other vegetables fall in the middle). But keep in mind, it's still better to eat those less nutritious vegetables than to munch on fat- and sugar-filled snacks, desserts, dairy, and meat.

VEGETABLES TO REMEMBER

Especially healthy ones	Less nutritious ones
Collard greens	Alfalfa sprouts
Spinach	Mushrooms
Kale	Eggplant
Swiss chard	Onions
Red pepper (raw)	Cucumber
Sweet potato (no skin)	Radishes
Pumpkin	Turnips
Carrots	Beets (canned)
Broccoli	Corn (frozen)
Okra	Iceberg lettuce

Source: Bonnie Liebman and Jayne Hurley, *Healthy Foods: Your Guide to the Best Basic Foods* (Washington, D. C.: Center for Science in the Public Interest, n.d.), pp. 8–9.

Vegetable superstars, such as sweet potatoes, spinach, and broccoli, can be dimmed if they're buried in butter and salt. Instead, season vegetables with lemon juice plus a sprinkle of oregano, an herb-spice mixture, basil or dill, or even nothing at all. On a baked potato, try low-fat margarine, low-fat sour cream, or salsa. Try low-fat salad dressing on steamed broccoli.

Start two new habits:

- Eat three half-cup servings of vegetables with every dinner.

- Try one new vegetable every week, such as steamed artichoke (with lemon juice), arugula, red or green cabbage, steamed kale, raw or sautéed rutabaga, or baked sweet potato (mush in crushed pineapple or applesauce).

8. CUT THE SALT

Salt is ubiquitous. Most of us became accustomed to salty foods in infancy, and continue eating salty processed foods all our lives. The sodium in salt increases the risk of high blood pressure—and that increases the risk of heart attack and stroke. Processed foods provide about 75 percent of the sodium in the average diet. After all, salt is much cheaper than flavorful natural ingredients.

The quickest way to cut back on sodium is to avoid processed foods (unless they are "low-salt" or "no-salt-added"). Canned or dried soups, frozen dinners, pizza, processed meats (hot dogs, ham, sausages), and processed cheeses are among the worst offenders. Check the Nutrition Facts label and buy the products that are lower in sodium.

Restaurants foods, too, are loaded with salt. And you often can't tell the sodium content by taste. For example, McDonald's sandwiches all have more sodium than the french fries. A Big Mac or Crispy Chicken sandwich has nearly half of an entire day's recommended daily intake of salt.

If you add salt to everything you eat, you should—today—replace your salt shaker with an herb shaker containing a commercial (e.g., Mrs. Dash's) or a homemade blend.

When you're cooking, replace salt with pepper, curry powder, salsa, mustard, and similar flavorful ingredients. Routinely use half as much (or less) salt as the recipe calls for. Keep lemon juice in a spray bottle in your refrigerator. Then you can easily spray your vegetables, fish, or other food, and add a sprinkle of herbs.

At first, dishes low in sodium may taste bland. But as your taste buds adjust, those "bland" foods begin to taste better and better.

9. MAKE FRUITS YOUR SNACKS

Eat plenty of fruit! Carry fruit as a snack. Eat it for dessert. Slice it into your cereal.

Fruit is naturally sweet and delicious—and often provides lots of vitamins A and C, folic acid, and other vitamins and minerals. Fruit also provides fiber and the phytochemicals that appear to reduce the risk of cancer, heart disease, and stroke.

A ready supply of fruit or fruit salad at home and at the office should ward off the temptation of junk foods in vending machines, snack bars, and fast-food restaurants. Dried apricots or dried fruit mixes are convenient ways to make sure a sweet snack is always at hand.

At breakfast, it takes just 60 seconds to peel an orange or section a grapefruit, or add lots of chopped fruit to your hot or cold whole grain cereal.

You should have fruit juice at home and at your workplace when you want more than water to quench your thirst. Orange and grapefruit juice are by far the most nutritious; apple and grape the least. Some juices now have calcium added to appeal to people (especially women) who need more calcium. To lighten up a juice and cut the calories, mix together equal portions of seltzer and juice, although it's better for children under five to stick with straight juice.

With the National Cancer Institute urging people to consume at least four or five servings of fruit each day, make sure that fruit is your morning or afternoon snack. Stock up now!

As with vegetables, some fruits are better than others. Below, we list nine particularly nutritious ones, along with those that rank lowest (with other fruits falling in the middle). But even the lowest-ranked fruits are a better dessert choice than chocolate brownies, cheesecake, or other calorie-laden, fat-filled foods.

FRUITS TO REMEMBER

Especially healthy ones	Less nutritious ones
Guava	Applesauce
Watermelon	Cranberry sauce (sweetened)
Grapefruit (pink)	Pears (canned)
Kiwifruit	Fruit cocktail
Papaya	Raisins
Cantaloupe	Dates (dried)
Apricots (dried)	Peaches (canned)
Orange	Prunes
Strawberries	Pineapple (canned)

Source: Liebman and Hurley, *Healthy Foods*, pp. 6–7.

Next time you're at a grocery store, seek out a few kinds of fruit that you never ate before. How about papaya, mango, star fruit, or unusual varieties of apples and pears?

10. AVOID SUGAR

Sugar (or corn syrup, dextrose, etc.) is a waste of calories, promotes obesity, causes tooth decay, and dilutes the nutritional quality of your diet.

Refined sugar is not a poison, and you don't have to eliminate it entirely. The problem is *excess*—which is what most Americans consume.

Soft drinks and other sugary beverages are the major source of sugar calories, and the problem has been getting worse as the size of the drinks increases. Coca-Cola was initially served in 6.5-ounce bottles, but then 12-ounce cans became standard. Over the past few years, 16- and 20-ounce bottles have started to become the norm, with fast-food restaurants serving even larger sizes. The 7-Eleven chain even sells a 64-ounce "Double Gulp."

A 12-ounce can is bad enough, in that it includes 10 teaspoons of sugar and 150 calories, but the Double Gulp features a mind-boggling 53 teaspoons of sugar and 800 calories. To help you kick the soft-drink habit, do an experiment and measure out onto a plate the 17 teaspoons of sugar in a 20-ounce soft-drink bottle. Then imagine eating all that sugar with a spoon at one sitting. You will likely feel sufficiently nauseated to throw your supersize soft drinks in the trash!

If you need any other incentives to cut down, consider that your body may not register the calories you *drink* as well as it does the calories you *eat.* So when you drink a soda or other high-calorie sugar beverage before or with a meal, you likely won't eat less food later in the day to compensate. In a study by Richard Mattes of Purdue University, people were asked to consume 450 calories of jelly beans every day for four weeks and 450 calories of soda every day for another four weeks. On the days they ate jelly beans, they compensated by eating 450 fewer calories over the course of the rest of the day. But when they drank the soda, they ended up eating roughly 450 more calories than usual. Other studies have shown a similar effect. As nutritionist Barbara Rolls of Pennyslvania State University points out, "The calories from most drinks add on to—rather than displace—food calories."[14]

What's even worse, soft drinks may increase the risk of osteoporosis by replacing milk, or the risk of cancer by replacing fruit juice. Therefore, drink water, fat-free milk, seltzer, or fruit juice instead of soft drinks.

You should also take an inventory of where you get your sugar. You can use the table on the next page. Once you know where your sugar intake comes from, start adjusting your diet. Leave sugar out of your tea or coffee. Switch to unsweetened cereals. Cut back on those fat-free, but hardly sugar-free, "healthy" frozen desserts, cookies, and cakes. Most important, cut back on ice cream, pies, chocolate, and other sweets that are loaded not just with sugar, but also fat. To satisfy your sweet tooth, eat fresh fruit, fruit salad, fruit juice, or fruit compote.

Artificial sweeteners don't have calories or cause tooth decay but might keep your sweet tooth alive. If you are going to use an artificial sweetener, choose sucralose (Splenda) or aspartame (NutraSweet and Equal), which seem to be the safest. Saccharin (Sweet 'N Low) and acesulfame-K (used in sugar-free gelatin desserts, syrups, etc.) may slightly increase your risk of cancer. Even aspartame might cause problems for some people. A tiny percentage of people who use it believe that it has caused dizziness, headaches, or epileptic-like seizures, but controlled studies have not yet substantiated any problems. Avoid it if you think you experience side effects, are pregnant, or suffer from PKU (phenylketonuria), a rare inability to metabolize the amino acid phenylalanine. Even if you don't have any of these conditions, to be safe, don't consume more than a couple of servings a day, and don't give it to infants.

SUGAR INVENTORY

Food	Servings per week
Soft drinks	_____
Cookies, cakes, pies, doughnuts	_____
Syrups and jams	_____
Fruit drinks (not 100% juice)	_____
Candy	_____
Ice cream, frozen yogurt, sherbet	_____
Sugar in coffee/tea	_____

AND IN ADDITION

Alcoholic Beverages

A drink (women) or two (men) a day may lower your risk of heart disease. But more than that becomes risky. If you do not drink, do not start. Exercising and eating better are much safer ways to improve your health.

Supplements

Even if you're eating a great diet, extra supplements make sense. Start with a multinutrient (like Centrum or a similar store brand) that has roughly 100 percent of the U.S. recommended Daily Value of 10 vitamins (A, B_1 [thiamin], B_2 [riboflavin], B_6, B_{12}, C, D, E, folic acid, and niacin) plus some vitamin K, along with the following mineral content: 100 percent of the Daily Value for zinc, copper, and chromium, plus some magnesium. If you're over 50, look for at least 25 micrograms of vitamin B_{12}. If you take a blood thinner like Coumadin, tell your doctor before taking any vitamin K. Women and children should consider taking some iron, and everyone can consider including some selenium.

Antioxidants may protect against chronic diseases. Consider taking daily 250 milligrams of vitamin C and 100 units of vitamin E. Adults (especially women) and teens (especially girls) should eat three or four servings of low-fat dairy products a day, or take 300 milligrams of calcium for every serving they skip.

If you may become pregnant, take a multivitamin that has 400 micrograms of folic acid (it's not good to wait until you are pregnant) to reduce the risk of birth defects. Folic acid also may fight heart disease in men and women.

On the other hand, don't overdo the supplements. Supplements are *not* an adequate substitute for a healthy diet. Moreover, taking too many vitamins and minerals can be harmful. The National Academy of Sciences recently established Tolerable Upper Intake Levels, or ULs, to indicate the safe upper limit for more than 20 nutrients. As Robert Russell, associate director of the Jean Mayer USDA Human Nutrition Research Center on Aging at Tufts University, notes, "Just going a little bit above the UL is not going to harm most people, but as you go higher and

---

GROWING AN APPRECIATION OF VEGETABLES

On Harvest Nights at the Kane Street Community Garden in LaCrosse, Wisconsin, low-income residents of the neighborhood come to the garden and help harvest the food. They take some of it home and donate the rest to food pantries. Sue Schultz of the LaCrosse Hunger Task Force, which started the garden, comes to the Harvest Nights to answer questions and to provide written information on the handling, storage, and cooking of the food. On evenings when an unusual item—such as kohlrabi—is harvested, she provides samples and recipes to the volunteers. Parents not only taste the samples themselves, but encourage their children to try the food. This translates into more vegetables eaten at home.

Harvest Nights are only one of many ways in which the Kane Street Community Garden brings improved nutrition, financial assistance, and a green oasis to the neighborhood. The garden is on a 1.8-acre piece of leased urban land. It is managed by a retired organic farmer and a garden coordinator who organize 200 volunteers and numerous activities at the garden. Volunteers receive a share of the 40,000

higher, you're increasing your risk of side effects."[15] Going over the UL on an occasional basis or under a doctor's supervision won't matter, but regular excessive use of supplements can cause mild effects like diarrhea or more serious damage. For example, excessive vitamin A from retinol can lead to severe liver disease and birth defects, yet health-food stores sell pills with more than twice the daily maximum upper limit. Too much zinc, niacin, vitamin D, or selenium can also cause significant problems. So don't go overboard.

Exercise

Although this book is about food choices, we would be remiss if we didn't end this chapter by emphasizing the importance of exercise. It helps you lose weight, strengthens the heart, and builds bones and muscle strength. Exercise also just makes you feel better. So build 30 minutes of exercise into your daily life: bike, walk, jog, garden, lift weights, play a sport. It is a critically important health habit.

pounds of organic produce that the garden yields throughout the season.

Schultz is not only the Hunger Task Force's president, an unpaid position; she's also a nutrition educator with the University of Wisconsin Cooperative Extension Service. So she helps provide education programs for the garden and evaluates the effectiveness of the project in delivering quality food, nutrition education, and a steady food supply to the neighborhood residents.

Twice a year the Hunger Task Force sponsors a Harvest Dinner at which meals are prepared using food from the garden and recipes are shared. The organization invites local officials to attend and uses the event to attract donations of supplies, equipment, and money.

All these activities have translated into a greater appreciation of fresh vegetables on the part of those in the neighborhood. A post-harvest survey after the 2000 growing season found that 94 percent of the participants in the project said they ate more vegetables because of their involvement with the garden. They also reported saving about $9 a week on their grocery bills when food was available from the garden.

CHAPTER SIX

THE FARMER'S NEW GENES: THE SAFETY OF BIOTECHNOLOGY

North American farmers have much to worry about, with low prices for the food they grow, variable weather, and cutthroat competition from competitors around the world. But now some of the farmers on the Canadian prairie have a new, unexpected concern: weeds created by genetic engineering.

In the spring of 2000, Lavern Affleck of Moosomin, Saskatchewan, started to notice genetically engineered canola plants sprouting up all over his wheat fields. When he talked to his neighbors, he discovered that they had the same problem.[1]

At first glance, this might not seem so surprising, since nearby farmers had planted the genetically modified canola, and it's common for seeds from one farm to be blown to another, where they plant themselves and sprout. The only catch is that in this case, the canola has been altered in a way that makes it hard to get rid of.

The biotechnology giant Monsanto Company had engineered the canola so that it was immune to the company's Roundup brand weed killer. The idea was that a farmer who planted Roundup-ready seeds could spray the herbicide on the field, killing all the weeds but not harming the canola. Farmers would be able to get rid of their weeds simply and inexpensively, thereby increasing their profits.

Once the genetically engineered canola gets into the fields of Affleck and his neighbors, they have a hard time removing it, since they can't use Roundup on it. As a result, they have to use a more expensive regime of several herbicides.

Although certainly a costly nuisance, the unwanted spread of canola in Saskatchewan is hardly the most serious environmental or economic problem facing farmers in Canada or the United States. Monsanto has even agreed to pay for any extra costs the wheat farmers incur to destroy the canola.

But what is most troubling is that many advocates of biotechnology had argued that a problem like Saskatchewan's could not possibly happen. According to them, anyone who alleged that genetically engineered plants would become hard-to-control weeds was an alarmist environmental extremist. They claimed that the new plants posed no different or more serious environmental threats than the many new plant varieties that are developed each year by traditional plant-breeding methods—methods that have been used for centuries.

As has become increasingly obvious to ecologists, genetically engineered plants bring some unique and troubling risks for the environment, including potential problems much more serious than canola weediness in Saskatchewan. The U.S. government—and indeed the world generally—needs a stronger, more effective set of regulatory practices to make sure that we can reap the benefits of biotechnology without causing serious harm to either humans or the environment.

But does this mean that consumers should avoid purchasing foods produced using biotechnology? Should you join the groups and individuals who call for a ban on genetically engineered foods, often denouncing them as "Frankenfoods"? Should you demand that the government place a moratorium on approvals of new genetically modified crops?

On balance, biotechnology is a powerful new tool whose upside outweighs its downside. Governments, scientists, biotechnology companies, farmers, and consumers can all help ensure that the helpful products of biotechnology get developed while the potentially harmful ones don't.

Unfortunately, opposition to genetically modified foods has been building, and there is a risk that consumers around the world will completely reject this new technology. This would be the same as if society banned computers because of destructive computer viruses and Internet porno sites. With biotechnology, as with computers, we need to find ways to minimize the problems while continuing to develop the technology.

This chapter provides background on the virtues and perils of genetically engineering foods. Then we will suggest a few ways to address genetically engineered foods—both at the supermarket and through the political process.

WHAT ARE GENETICALLY MODIFIED FOODS AND WHY WOULD ANYONE WANT TO PRODUCE THEM?

Let's start by defining the term "biotechnology." Biotechnology refers to any "use of biological processes for the development of products such as foods, enzymes, drugs, and vaccines."[2] Without using the word, people engaged in biotechnology for thousands of years when they made cheese, wine, and other fermented foods. But, more recently, popular use of the term "biotechnology" has been associated with efforts to genetically modify, or "engineer," organisms.

All plants, animals, and bacteria contain deoxyribonucleic acid (DNA), molecules whose particular arrangement constitutes the genetic makeup of those organisms. Little segments of DNA, called genes, convey specific characteristics to the organism. An animal or plant might have 25,000 different genes, or even more. Some genes control the color of a plant; some determine the size and shape of an animal; others influence the personality of a person. Starting in the 1970s, scientists devised ways to identify and isolate a specific gene from an organism and insert it into another. Since the DNA code is essentially universal, the transferred gene can often function in the new organism in which it is placed. Although the methods of genetic engineering were initially laborious and limiting, both scientists and financial investors understood the long-term potential of the technology. Billions of dollars were quickly invested in biotechnology companies.

The two largest uses of genetically modified organisms are for medicines and foods. As early as 1978, a company called Genentech genetically engineered human insulin, and now most insulin-dependent diabetics rely on that product of biotechnology. Genetic engineering has also produced human growth hormone and other medical products that improve people's quality of life and generate little controversy.[3]

Genetically engineered crops took longer to develop, and the first ones were planted in the early 1990s. Although farmers have been gradually altering plants for thousands of years—just compare a modern corn or potato plant with its wild relatives—genetic engineering gives scientists the ability to produce new types of organisms that they couldn't possibly produce through long-established processes such as crossbreeding.

For example, a gene can be taken from a broccoli plant or bacterium and inserted into a potato plant to make a new, genetically modified type of potato. Even more dramatically, a fish or a fox gene can be inserted into a lettuce plant.

At least for the near future, this won't lead to all sorts of Frankenstein monsters, since scientists can only insert one or a few genes at a time. This means that the resulting plant remains almost the same as the original version, with virtually all of its thousands of genes unaltered, although some unpredictable changes can occur.

From the early to the late 1990s, the amount of land given over to genetically modified crops—especially corn, cotton, and soybeans—skyrocketed. In the United States, where most genetically engineered crops are grown, the number of acres planted went from just 3 million in 1996 to 71 million in 1999. The sales of genetically engineered crops generated more than $2 billion in the latter year.[4] The public was barely aware of this development because most of the early engineered crops incorporated changes that were of value to farmers but invisible to consumers.

In the future, genetically modified foods should also provide consumers with significant benefits, assuming that the technology is allowed to develop. In the summer of 2000, leaders from the national academies of science in the United States, Britain, China, India, Brazil, and other countries issued a report on the potential of biotechnology in agriculture. They concluded that it can and "should be used to increase the production of main food staples, improve the efficiency of production, reduce the environmental impacts of agriculture, and provide access to food for small-scale farmers."[5]

We can divide the potential benefits of genetically engineered foods into five main categories: higher yields, lower environmental impacts, ability to grow food in more places, more healthful foods, and protection for valuable crops.

1. Higher Yields

For generations, farmers, with the help of scientists, have been improving their practices to produce more food on a given amount of land. Two simple mathematical facts—the world's population is growing rapidly, but the amount of land remains constant—make it essential that the trend toward higher yields continues. Biotechnology can help achieve that, but traditional plant breeding and other technologies are equally important.

As just one example, scientists in Kenya and the United States are developing a virus-resistant sweet potato that has increased yields more than 20 percent in field trials.[6] That is not only good news for the global food supply, but should be good economic news for farmers and the environment. If we can produce more food per acre, less natural habitat will need to be devoted to agricultural uses.

In the past, some yield increases—those based on the use of toxic pesticides and nitrogen-rich fertilizers—have had huge environmental costs. But genetic engineering offers the possibility of increasing yields without increasing these sorts of inputs.

The need to produce more food for their growing populations has led China and India to invest significant national funds into biotechnology. Chinese scientists, for example, are creating a rice variety that produces twice as many rice kernels per stalk. The use of insect-resistant cotton in China has boosted yields while reducing harm to wildlife from insecticides.[7]

2. Lower Environmental Impacts

In addition to increasing farmers' yields, there are other ways in which genetic engineering can benefit the environment. The USDA's Economic Research Service estimates that genetic engineering cut the quantity of active pesticide ingredients used by more than 1.0 million pounds between 1997 and 1998. Some studies of specific crops have shown a similar trend. For example, even though herbicide-tolerant soybeans haven't reduced total pesticide use, they have decreased the number of times pesticides are applied and led to a shift to safer herbicides. Insect-resistant cotton, although not a food crop, reduced insecticide use significantly while increasing yields. Some of the positive results could be short lived if pests develop resistance to the genetically engineered crops.[8] But as scientists learn more about the performance of genetically engineered crops, they should be able to develop new varieties that produce assured reductions in pesticide use.

Another major benefit of the widely planted herbicide-tolerant soybeans is that many farmers don't need to plow their fields to kill weeds. That reduces soil erosion and water pollution associated with tilling.[9]

3. Ability to Grow Food in More Places

If farmers could better use lands currently poorly suited to agriculture, they could produce considerably more food. To accomplish this, scientists are working on a wide range of genetically engineered crops that could withstand various stresses, such as drought, salt, cold, or periodic flooding. For example, scientists at the University of Delhi in India have produced a rice variety that can survive prolonged submergence under water, a common occurrence in Bangladesh and India. It will be three or four more years before the first stress-tolerant plant—probably a cold-resistant canola being developed for use in Canada—is grown on a commercial scale.[10]

As we will see, there may be environmental risks from these sorts of crops. But as long as they are introduced and monitored carefully, they should provide great benefit in the coming era of increasing population and decreasing availability of good farm land.

4. More Healthful Foods

The biotech industry has long touted the possibility of more nutritious, safer food. Companies are developing soy, corn, and canola plants that will produce oils lower in artery-clogging saturated fats. They are also developing potatoes that will absorb less oil when fried. These sorts of plants will look and act very similar to current varieties but will be somewhat healthier to eat. For the most part, though, benefits to consumers are years away.

More important will be plants with enhanced levels of vitamins and minerals—the so-called micronutrients. Many people around the world currently subsist on a limited, unvarying diet that provides insufficient vitamins and minerals. In fact, at least 20 percent of the world's population gets too few micronutrients. And they can't afford vitamin supplements. Scientists are therefore using genetic engineering and other methods to develop plants with higher levels of the missing nu-trients.

The first major genetically modified food to be developed for its higher micronutrient levels is called "golden rice," because of its light, golden-yellow color. It has been engineered to include beta-carotene, which is converted to vitamin A in humans. Because 80 million children around the world suffer from vitamin A deficiency, which can lead to blindness or even death, golden rice has great promise. In Asia, many poor children subsist on rice gruel and the new rice could help them to get more vitamin A. Similarly, rice that is engineered to have higher lev-els of iron could help the nearly 2 billion people who suffer from anemia because of iron deficiency.[11]

If you think about biotechnology's potential, the total ban on engi-neered food that some critics advocate seems shortsighted and unfair to the world's poor. Hassan Adamu, Nigeria's minister of agricultural and rural development, complains that "to deny desperate, hungry people the means to control their futures by presuming to know what is best for them is not only paternalistic, but morally wrong." The United Nations Development Programme, which focuses on helping improve the lives of people in developing countries, has concluded that biotechnology can "drive the development of new crop varieties with greater drought and disease resistance, less environmental stress and more nutritional value. Biotechnology offers the only or the best 'tool of choice' for marginal ecological zones—left behind by the green revolution but home to more than half of the world's poorest people, dependent on agriculture and livestock."[12]

Nevertheless, we shouldn't exaggerate the potential benefits of the initial micronutrient-enhanced crops. "Golden" crops will have to pro-vide high enough levels of nutrients to be useful, and their appearance and taste will have to be acceptable. The current variety of golden rice does not provide enough B-carotene to eliminate Vitamin A deficiency. Golden rice alone would therefore make only a modest dent in malnutrition-related diseases and would work best as just one part of a comprehensive strategy for addressing hunger and poverty.

The biotech industry has overhyped golden rice in an effort to win public support and to show that it cares about more than profits. Given that golden rice was funded by the Rockefeller Foundation rather than any biotech company, the industry campaign has been especially self-serving, but it shouldn't prevent us from seeing the indisputable fact that biotechnology could produce healthier foods.

5. Protection for Valuable Crops

Some food crops are extremely vunerable to disease. Just take the case of bananas. The banana industry currently relies on only a couple of varieties. If a new, incurable disease were to appear, all the world's commercial banana plants could be killed. In fact, a fungus wiped out many banana farms in the 1940s and 1950s, and the only thing that al-lowed the industry to recover was the discovery in Vietnam of a variety of banana resistant to the fungus. The next time farmers may not be so lucky as to find a naturally occurring strain that could resist a new dis-ease, but genetic engineering could be used to develop such a resistant variety.[13]

In Hawaii, papaya trees have long been subject to the tree-killing papaya ring spot virus. Once this disease attacks a plantation, there is nothing that can be done to stop its deadly progress. In fact, the disease has wiped out all the commercial papaya trees on the island of Oahu, which used to be a major papaya-growing region. To deal with this prob-lem, Dennis Gonsalves, a scientist at Cornell University, worked with colleagues at other institutions to develop a genetically modified variety of papaya whose fruit looks, feels, and tastes the same as conventional papaya but is not susceptible to the virus.[14] That engineered variety of papaya is saving the Hawaiian papaya industry and similar varieties are starting to be grown in Southeast Asia.

THE GROWING OPPOSITION TO GENETICALLY MODIFIED FOODS

Given biotechnology's ability to provide us with healthier food at a lower environmental cost, why have increasing numbers of people op-posed it? In great part, the biotechnology industry has brought this problem on itself. Not only did the industry commercialize the technology extremely fast, but it presented new products to the public—especially in Europe—in arrogant, insensitive ways virtually guaranteed to build mistrust and skepticism. The industry also fell victim to some bad luck and silly mistakes.

Right from the start, the advocates of genetically engineered foods painted an unrealistic picture of the technology that exaggerated its potential benefits and dismissed its risks. When some of their overly rosy statements were later proven wrong, the companies—and, by extension, the technology—seemed to be unworthy of the public's trust.

Whether it be robots, computers, or genetically modified foods, the early developers of a new technology often fall into hyperbole and exaggeration. They get caught up in their enthusiasm for their new invention and optimistically spin scenarios that present it as a panacea. Rather than acknowledge the modest initial social contribution biotechnology could make, its advocates promoted a utopian vision in which it would "feed the world," ending food shortages and hunger. The companies envisioned making profits while simultaneously saving society. Molecular biologists, excited by their ever-expanding ability to understand the genetic structure of living organisms, took comfort from believing that they were not only advancing their professional careers, but were solving vexing global problems. They didn't, however, try to understand the causes of world hunger, and they downplayed the potential dangers of biotechnology.

As we have seen, biotechnology can be an important tool to help increase the planet's food supply, but it doesn't provide much of an answer to world hunger in the short run. The biotech companies have unsurprisingly focused their research on endeavors that can yield sales to paying customers—and there are many more potential paying customers in affluent countries than poor ones. Hence companies have developed varieties of corn, cotton, and soybeans adapted for use in developed countries rather than rice, cassaua, cowpeas, and other crops grown in the developing nations of Africa, Asia, and Latin America.

Nevertheless, the handy assertion that biotechnology would feed the world allowed its proponents to cloak themselves in altruism and attack their critics for trying to delay the implementation of a lifesaving technology. "Feeding the world" remained a largely unexamined mantra until the ranks of biotechnology's critics became so numerous in the late 1990s that they placed the industry on the defensive.

One thing that strengthened and emboldened biotechnology's opponents was clear evidence that the industry and government officials had ignored or intentionally downplayed the risks of genetically engineered crops. Back in the 1980s, the young biotechnology companies asserted that genetically modified plants posed no different or greater risks to the environment or human health than did the many new products that traditional breeding practices brought to grocery shelves each year. They claimed that biotechnology just represented a faster, more accurate way to develop new plants. With biotechnology research costing billions of dollars, industry leaders were anxious to get their products to market.

Scientists working on genetic engineering downplayed the risks of biotechnology for a different reason. They were molecular biologists who operated in laboratories and thought about one type of organism at a time. They felt confident that they understood what they were producing and that their lab tests could ensure the safety of any new foods. In terms of food safety, they were generally right. The most notable exception was the insertion of an allergy-causing protein from Brazil nuts into soybeans. However, the company, Pioneer Hi-Bred International, figured out the problem through follow-up lab testing and never marketed that variety of soybean.[15]

But the molecular biologists had less understanding of how new organisms would interact with existing life-forms in complex environments outside of the lab. Most ecologists—those scientists who specialize in studying how various plants and animals interact in the real world—initially gave little attention to biotechnology, but later began to express concerns about the technology's risks. In the late 1980s and early 1990s, only a handful of ecologists and a few scientists at the environmental organizations Environmental Defense Fund and Union of Concerned Scientists argued that government regulations needed to be strengthened.

But even without any environmental catastrophes, the industry inflicted several public relations disasters on itself. The first was caused by not developing products that consumers would see as beneficial because they either taste better, are healthier, or last longer. Even though the industry's widely distributed publicity materials promised that biotechnology would give consumers tastier, cheaper, and more nutritious foods, its initial products (with one or two exceptions) benefited only farmers—by controlling insects, weeds, or plant diseases. In part, that was because those products were the easiest ones to engineer. But it also reflected the biotech companies' determination that they could make the quickest profits by appealing to the needs of farmers rather than the desires of consumers. Although sales figures exploded, the public wasn't given any reason to value biotechnology. When some of its potential risks started to become apparent, some activists called for a ban on it since they saw it as something that wasn't benefiting them, but could potentially harm their health or the environment.

The most publicized effort in the United States to show that genetic engineering could produce something consumers would desire—the Calgene Flavr Savr tomato—was an embarrassing flop. The Calgene company started with the premise that fruit that ripens on the vine tastes better. They therefore engineered a tomato that could be left longer on the vine, yet would still be firm enough to ship to market without damage. William Hiatt, the company's director of tomato research, promised

---

GOT (ENGINEERED) MILK?

When, in 1994, many of the nation's cows started receiving injections of a Monsanto product named Posilac, large numbers of Americans began for the first time to consume food produced with genetic engineering. Posilac is a laboratory-produced version of a protein called bovine somatotropin (BST), or bovine growth hormone (BGH), that cows produce naturally to regulate their milk production. When cows are injected with Posilac, their milk production goes up 10 percent or more. Today, about one-third of America's milk cows receive it.

The FDA, the UN's Joint Expert Committee on Food Additives, and various medical journals have concluded that milk from these cows is perfectly safe for humans. It has essentially the same flavor, appearance, nutritional value, and chemical composition as milk from cows that haven't received BGH supplements. The milk from the

that "once they're in the supermarket, they will soften normally," and that they would stay fresh nearly twice as long as other breeds. Calgene spent $20 million and eight years to develop and field-test its tomato. Food-safety experts gave it a clean bill of health. The Flavr Savr seemed "tailor-made to convince the public that biotech food is safe as spinach," according to one commentator. Calgene was so confident of the superiority of its tomato that it predicted consumers would make 15 percent of their tomato purchases Flavr Savrs, even though it carried a much higher price tag than average tomatoes.[16]

Unfortunately for Calgene, its tomato turned out to be less firm than expected and was hard to ship and distribute without bruising. On top of that, consumers didn't think it tasted any better than other much cheaper tomatoes. And it faced competition from improved tomato strains bred by traditional methods. The Calgene company suffered financially and was taken over by Monsanto, which discontinued the Flavr Savr.[17] With the demise of the Flavr Savr, there is still no genetically engineered food that offers consumers a perceived benefit.

Nevertheless, the biotechnology industry kept growing in the United States as more farmers planted crops that promised them in-

---

Posilac-treated cows has slightly higher amounts of insulin growth factor 1 (IGF-1) than it would otherwise, but the increase is less than the variations that occur naturally between the milk of different cows or even in the milk from the same cow at different times.

Although there's no evidence that the IGF-1 levels in milk—either from BGH-treated or other cows—is harmful, more research is needed, and scientists should continue to investigate its potential impacts. But even if it eventually turns out that IGF-1 is a problem, it is highly unlikely that drinking the small extra amount of IGF-1 in milk from BGH-treated cows would significantly increase your risk of illness.

Posilac has been controversial ever since it came on the market. Canada and the European Union have not permitted its sale. Some of the opposition comes from people who object to all genetic engineering. But some of it stems from the fact that Posilac injections increase the risk of mastitis infections and other health problems in cows.

creased profits. In 1999, half of the soybeans, one-third of the corn, and nearly half of the cotton grown were genetically engineered. But in that year, genetic engineering was undercut from several directions. Growing opposition in Europe made headlines and led farmers, processors, retailers, and consumers to reject engineered crops and foods. Also, mad cow disease and other food-safety concerns totally unconnected to genetic engineering had convinced many people—especially in England—that the food supply was increasingly unsafe and that governments were either unwilling or unable to do anything about it. Having lost faith in government regulators and multinational food companies, many European consumers didn't trust assurances that genetically engineered foods were risk-free. And activists at Greenpeace and other groups pressured grocery stores and food processors to reject foods containing genetically engineered ingredients.

In England, many public figures, including the Prince of Wales, fueled the opposition. The prince wrote a widely quoted article in 1999 in the *Daily Telegraph* charging that genetically modified food "takes mankind into realms that belong to God, and to God alone. . . . I personally have no wish to eat anything produced by genetic modification, nor do I knowingly offer this sort of produce to my family or guests." By the start of the new millenium, only 25 percent of England's population wanted to encourage "use of biotechnology to produce foods," while 42 percent was opposed and 33 percent was unsure.[18]

POISONED BUTTERFLIES AND TAINTED TACO SHELLS

As public opposition to biotechnology was growing in Europe, the biotechnology industry faced a domestic public relations nightmare in the United States. In May 1999, Cornell University scientists published a study based on a laboratory experiment in which monarch butterfly caterpillars died after they ate milkweed leaves covered with pollen from genetically engineered corn plants. On one level, this wasn't surprising since the corn was designed to be toxic to the European corn borer, a close relative of monarch butterflies. Any insecticide targeted at a particular pest will likely also harm related insects. The experiment led to a firestorm of publicity as critics used the beloved butterfly as a symbol of the risks of biotechnology. In the wake of the Cornell study and until scientists could determine whether the butterflies are actually vulnerable in cornfields, the Environmental Protection Agency asked farmers to take precautions to protect the monarch butterflies.[19]

Since then, studies published in the September 2001 *Proceedings of the National Academy of Sciences* demonstrated that the threat to the butterflies was most likely negligible, but that won't undo the damage to the reputation of the biotechnology industry.

In the wake of the butterfly fiasco and the European backlash, some biotechnology leaders realized that they needed to back off from their often arrogant public posture. Charles Holliday Jr., DuPont's chief executive, admitted that "public concern has been aggravated by the perception that we in industry have often acted as though public fears are not legitimate and are the result of ignorance. But we have to listen to the people who are now raising alarms." The head of Monsanto, Robert Shapiro, admitted that his company had been guilty of "condescension or indeed arrogance" and needed to change its approach.[20]

Nevertheless, much damage to the industry had already been done. A coalition of 30 farm groups warned their members that planting genetically modified crops would put them at financial risk.[21]

The year 2000 brought the industry's most expensive blunder, the taco shell debacle. On September 17, Genetically Engineered Food Alert, a coalition of public interest groups opposed to biotechnology, announced that it had discovered traces of genetically engineered StarLink brand corn in Taco Bell taco shells. Aventis CropSciences, the developer of the corn, had received government approval for feeding it to livestock and for industrial uses such as producing ethanol. Because there was a chance that the pesticidal protein engineered into the corn might cause allergic reactions when ingested, the government did not approve it for the food supply. But now it was turning up in human food.

Aventis apparently never took seriously the possibility that its corn might contaminate human food. Even strenuous efforts might not have prevented contamination, but Aventis gave farmers precious little information and no compelling reason to keep the special corn separate. When later investigating how the corn ended up in tacos, company officials found that some of the farmers who had bought the StarLink corn did not know it wasn't approved for human consumption, while others had forgotten about this restriction.[22]

Aventis and the USDA had to mount a costly search for all products containing the corn. The Mission Foods company alone had to recall 300 varieties of taco shells, tortillas, and snack chips sold in restaurants like Applebee's and under supermarket brand names including Kroger, Safeway, and Wal-Mart. Some consumers temporarily avoided all tacos. Even though the StarLink corn had been planted on less than half of 1 percent of the corn acres in the country, the USDA ultimately found traces of it in 9 percent of the more than 100,000 batches of corn it tested.[23]

Not only did the taco debacle cost food companies million of dollars and send Aventis's stock into a tailspin, but, for many Americans who did not have firm views on genetically engineered foods, it created the impression that the technology was risky. It also demonstrated the inade-

---

REMEMBERING THE WORLD'S POOR

In recent years, Per Pinstrup-Andersen has tried to remind Americans opposing biotechnology of the needs of 800 million people around the world who go to bed hungry. Pinstrup-Andersen is completing his second five-year term as director-general of the Washington-based International Food Policy Research Institute, the key international agency carrying out policy analysis on ways to sustainably improve food production in the developing world. His agency has traditionally focused on technical studies for government officials and agricultural researchers, but he has increasingly urged the United States and Europe not to prevent poor countries from using biotechnology.

Many people in developing countries spend more than half their disposable income on food (compared to 10 percent for Americans), yet they still can't afford an adequate diet. They have an urgent need for better, cheaper food, and biotechnology could help provide it. Pinstrup-Andersen recognizes fully that biotechnology alone won't end hunger and poverty, but he argues that any technology that has the potential to make a dent in the massive problem of malnutrition should be made available to developing countries.

quacy of government oversight. The FDA was shown to have no procedure in place for monitoring contamination, and only investigation by a private environmental group uncovered the StarLink problem.

Even the most gung ho biotech advocates worried about fallout from the taco episode. As Sano Shomoda of the biotech investment firm BioScience Securities admitted, "This relatively small incident, in terms of acreage, has turned into a multiheaded monster. There's going to be a backlash on multiple fronts. It's going to fundamentally delay growth in the development of this technology."[24]

Indeed, over the past two years, the introduction of new genetically engineered crops has slowed. Food processors are concerned about their export markets in light of the increasingly intense opposition on the part of European consumers, who view biotechnology as one of many misguided efforts by the United States to unilaterally impose its view of the world on Europe. Sensibly, American food companies and some farmers have concluded that they shouldn't march forward too fast with genetic

---

Although biotechnology certainly has risks—and appropriate precautions need to be taken—Pinstrup-Andersen wants us to compare those risks to the potentially serious human health costs of preventing its implementation in the developing world. He observes, "Condemning agricultural biotechnology for its potential risks without considering the alternative risks of prolonging the human misery caused by hunger, malnutrition, and child death is as unwise and unethical as blindly pursuing this technology without the necessary safety measures." With 5 million preschool children dying each year from nutrition-related causes, even a partial solution to malnutrition would save and improve large numbers of lives.

On the other hand, Pinstrup-Andersen isn't a big fan of the biotech companies and doesn't expect them to give much attention to the world's poor, despite their rhetoric about biotechnology "feeding the world." There just isn't enough money in it for them. He has therefore urged governments, foundations, and international development agencies to invest much more heavily in biotech and other research aimed specifically at producing crops that would increase the productivity of small farms in poor countries and improve the nutrition of poor people.

engineering until their overseas customers have accepted engineered foods.

The biotech companies have also realized that the increasingly complex global trade routes of food products have made it more costly and complicated to introduce genetically engineered foods into the market. Debi Warnick of Syngenta Seeds points out that her company raises melon seeds in Asia. The melons are then grown in Central America and shipped to the United States for sale. Any genetically engineered melon seeds would need to receive regulatory approval from at least three countries. So Syngenta will forego commercializing genetically engineered melons, at least until the path to regulatory approval becomes clearer and easier.[25]

For the moment, the big biotechnology companies are focusing on just a few big crops that have genetically engineered varieties already on sale. American farmers continue to plant those varieties on more acres—88 million in 2001.[26] But the controversy over biotechnology has slowed down an industry that was moving too fast and making costly mistakes.

RISKS OF GENETICALLY ENGINEERED FOODS

Now that the biotechnology juggernaut has been slowed, it is important to ensure that society doesn't overreact and stop genetic engineering altogether, as some of its opponents would like. Biotechnology still has the potential to provide us with a more healthful, abundant, and environmentally friendly food supply.

Although the genetic engineering of food may entail risks, we need to keep in mind that our current food system already causes serious problems for the environment and public health. Americans need to assess whether the environment and public health would be better off with or without biotechnology. On balance, genetically engineered food will provide many benefits as long as governments develop meaningful regulations and consumers remain vigilant. Strong government regulation is the best route to winning consumer support and preventing environmental or health problems.

In April 2000, a team of distinguished scientists appointed by the National Research Council, the research wing of the National Academy of Sciences, issued a report on the science and regulation of genetically modified plants. While pointing out the need for stronger government oversight, the committee "emphasized it was not aware of any evidence suggesting foods on the market today are unsafe to eat as a result of genetic modification."[27]

One important health risk biotechnology developers need to avoid is the introduction of new allergens into the food supply. Scientists have the ability to test for known food allergens and the genes that code for them. They can also guard against engineered foods with dangerous levels of known naturally occurring toxins, such as solanine in potatoes.

It is harder to guard against food allergies that might be caused by the use of genes from bacteria or plants that haven't previously been consumed as food. Scientists have studied known food allergens to understand what it is about them that causes reactions. They have learned that food allergens tend to be of a certain molecular size and to be relatively resistant to acids and heat. But scientists need to develop better methods for identifying potential allergens—not just in genetically engineered foods, but generally.

The greater risks from genetically modified crops are not to human health, but to the environment. The risks fall into four categories: the new plants could become weeds, their pollen could mix with wild relatives to produce weeds, they could lead to hard-to-control insect pests, and, perhaps most worrisome, they could cause some unexpected problem. In addition, genetically engineered fish pose some special concerns.

1. Genetically Engineered Plants Could Become Weeds

Simply defined, weeds "are plants that happen to be in the wrong place at the wrong time. Indeed no plant is intrinsically a weed. . . . [T]he same plant may be a weed in one situation and a desirable plant (such as a crop or lawn grass) in another."[28] To Saskatchewan farmer Lavern Affleck, who we met at the beginning of this chapter, the genetically engineered canola plants sprouting up in his fields are weeds, but they are valuable crops to the farmers who intentionally planted them.

Many serious weed problems have been caused over the past 100 years by plant species—like kudzu or purple loosestrife—that were transferred from one part of the world to another. Cornell University entomologist David Pimentel estimates that these sorts of "invasive species" cost American society $137 billion a year and that "128 species of plants intentionally introduced as crops have become serious weeds."[29]

Changing only one or two genes in an ordinarily unproblematic plant, like corn or potatoes, is very unlikely to cause a weed problem outside the agricultural environment. Some biotech advocates have therefore argued to government regulators that the weediness potential should be ignored. Any problems from biotechnology are unlikely to be as serious as the traditional route to an out-of-control invasive species—bringing a plant from some other country into the United States—and those sorts of transfers are only weakly regulated. Such arguments seem seriously misguided since there is still some risk from biotechnology. Instead of failing to control biotechnology because other types of plants are poorly regulated, the government should strengthen both types of regulations.[30]

Plants engineered to tolerate stresses, like drought, cold, and salt, are, by definition, able to survive in additional locations and thereby more likely to become weeds. Although most crop plants have traits that make them uncompetitive in nonfarm habitats, it is important that the government review new products to ensure that plants with increased survival traits do not threaten wild habitats. As with the other risks of genetically modified crops, this potential problem could be controlled by taking adequate precautions, but it shouldn't be ignored.

2. Genetically Engineered Plants Could Mix with Other Plants in Undesirable Ways

If farmers plant a crop near sexually compatible wild relatives, it's almost inevitable that some pollen will be transferred to those relatives. If the resulting plant now has a characteristic that makes it more likely to survive, such as cold or drought tolerance, that plant could outcompete its neighbors and alter the wild ecosystem. Before a genetically engineered plant is grown in a particular location, scientists need to assess whether any wild relatives are nearby. A genetically engineered corn plant that could be safely grown in Massachusetts might not be safe in parts of Mexico where teosinte, the ancestor of corn, grows near farmers' fields.

The USDA took an unnecessary risk in the mid-1990s when, despite limited testing and concerns expressed by many scientists and environmental groups, it allowed genetically engineered virus-resistant squashes to be grown near wild relatives. Even though the USDA admitted that the new squash could pass on its genes to its wild relatives, the agency claimed there was little chance of creating troublesome weeds.[31] When a committee sponsored by the National Academy of Sciences later studied the issue, it chastised the USDA, saying the agency's position was "not well supported by scientific studies."[32] Biotech companies and the government need to be more careful in the future.

Another problem could occur if the pollen from certain genetically engineered crops ends up in the fields of organic farmers, transferred there by birds, insects, and the wind. This sort of "pollen drift" has turned out to be much more widespread than scientists anticipated. In the case of Minnesota organic corn farmers Susan and Mark Fitzgerald, they bought corn seeds guaranteed to be biotechnology free. Yet, because of drifting pollen from other farms, some of their corn turned out to be contaminated with so much genetically engineered corn kernels that they couldn't sell it as organic. They had to reduce the price on 800 bushels, losing nearly $2,000.[33] The courts will end up deciding whether biotech companies have to pay organic farmers for such economic losses, but the bigger issue is how to ensure that organic farmers can continue to produce crops substantially free of this type of genetic material. (Foods can contain small amounts of pesticides and engineered genes and still be considered organic.) Most organic farmers are not seriously threatened by pollen drift, but precautions need to be taken to protect as many of the remaining ones as possible, especially if biotech fruits and vegetables are marketed.

3. Genetically Engineered Plants Could Lead to Hard-to-Control Insect Pests

One of the most popular types of genetically modified plants on the market is the so-called Bt plant. *Bacillus thuringiensis* (Bt) is a naturally occurring bacterium that organic farmers and gardeners have long used to control various insect pests. Various strains of that bacterium produce proteins that are lethal to several kinds of insects. That protein is much safer than most chemical pesticides. For this reason, scientists engineered the Bt into corn, cotton, and potato plants so that they would naturally and safely keep away harmful pests.

The only catch is that if strict precautions aren't taken, the insects can, over time, develop resistance to Bt. The genetically engineered plants would lose their insecticidal powers and the bacterium would no longer work for organic farmers. That would be a special tragedy for organic farmers who have few alternatives to Bt.

Environmentalists and ecologists warned about this problem early on, but the biotech companies and the Environmental Protection Agency downplayed the concern and took only weak protective measures. In the meantime, the number of acres planted with Bt crops increased to over 9 million in 1997. Evidence mounted that the environmentalists were right, and then the National Academy of Sciences weighed in, finding that the EPA's policies were insufficient to prevent insect resistance.[34] Finally the EPA admitted the need for stronger regulations, intensified its research efforts, and began to require corn farmers to plant some of their fields with non-Bt crops. The idea is that nonresistant insects will flourish in the non-Bt fields and would breed with any resistant ones, diluting the resistance. Nevertheless, more than a quarter of the farmers who grow Bt crops may not be complying fully with the rules. Moreover, even under the best of circumstances, the precautions are not guaranteed to work indefinitely.

4. Unexpected Problems

Ecologists realize that complex ecosystems with many different plants, animals, bacteria, soils, rocks, and minerals are notoriously hard to understand. As biotech crops are planted on millions of acres, something could happen that scientists never expected. As Chris Hables Gray, a scholar of the relationship between science and society, warned the National Research Council, "our ability to fully understand and predict the future of complex systems is quite limited. . . . No doubt many of the scientists working in the area of transgenic research [biotechnology] will confidently claim that they know all the possible ramifications of what they are doing. Please don't believe them."[35]

Scientists will have a hard time predicting the possible ramifications of growing novel crops on a large scale in new places. What would it mean for indigenous bird, mammal, and insect populations if farmers were to start growing cold-resistant rice in Minnesota? Could local weather patterns be affected by wide-scale planting of drought-resistant crops in arid areas? Down the road, there could also be some sort of un-expected toxicity or other food-safety effect from a particular genetically engineered food.[36]

The chance that there could be unwelcome surprises should not halt the development of genetic engineering, but it should make scientists, biotech company executives, farmers, policymakers, and consumers cautious. It should also spur greater investment in studying potential environmental implications of genetically engineered crops. Up to now, less than 5 percent of the USDA's research budget on biotechnology has gone to assessing environmental risks.[37]

5. Fish: A Special Case

As more of the fish that people eat gets raised on farms, some biotechnology advocates have embraced the idea of modifying fish so that those farms could be more productive. That is similar to the idea of increasing the yield on land-based farms that grow plants.

But there is one big difference. If genetically engineered fish are raised on a large scale, it is highly likely that some of those fish will escape and breed with native species. Fish farms have been notoriously prone to fish escapes and, unless special precautions are taken, there's no reason to believe that fish farms with genetically engineered fish would be any different. When fish and other sea animals are introduced into new environments, they can wreak havoc. In perhaps the most infamous case, zebra mussels that found their way into the Great Lakes have caused billions of dollars worth of damage by clinging to metal surfaces, clogging water intakes and treatment systems. In a different case, before the Nile perch was introduced into Lake Victoria in Africa in the 1950s, there were 500 native species of fish. Today, most of them—including catfish, lungfish, and tilapia—have been decimated, and local fishermen are only able to catch 3 native species in useful quantities.[38]

Aqua Bounty Farms is developing a genetically engineered fish—a type of salmon that can reach marketable size in less than half the time required by conventional farm-raised salmon, and with a 20 percent reduction in feed. Other types of fish are being engineered to grow faster or survive in colder water. But these are exactly the sorts of changes that could allow engineered fish to outcompete wild ones and thereby dramatically change aquatic ecosystems. Even if the engineered fish turn out to be less hardy than conventional ones in the wild, it could still be a problem. Two Purdue University biologists have sketched a scenario in which fast-growing, larger-than-normal engineered male fish would be very successful at mating with wild females. The offspring would be less able to survive in the wild, thereby making the overall stock of the species weaker.[39]

BRINGING SCIENCE TO THE TABLE

By planting genetically engineered crops on millions of acres, Americans are, in effect, conducting a massive experiment. But it's not easy for scientists to figure out how the experiment is going or what all the environmental risks are.

To get a better handle on these issues, Kim Waddell, a program officer in the research arm of the National Academy of Sciences, works with leading scientists from around the world. They try to look beyond the heated rhetoric and emotional debate over genetic engineering to dispassionately assess its potential environmental and health consequences. They then advise the federal government on how it should monitor and regulate biotechnology.

Up to now, there has been relatively little funding for studying the impacts of transgenic crops, something Waddell would like to see changed. But many other food-related subjects deserve further study as well. "There's a lot scientists still don't understand about agriculture," Waddell points out, "for example, what's going on below ground with the communities of microorganisms that live in the soil. We're just beginning to identify many of the species, let alone figure out how they might affect agricultural production." One of the National Academy's most important tasks, therefore, is to define the types of scientific

Because of the probability of escapes from fish farms, considerable research into the risks of a particular genetically engineered fish variety needs to be done before government officials approve any such fish, and careful precautions should be taken after any approval. Unfortunately, the federal government is currently poorly positioned to insist on such measures, in great part because the current environmental laws did not foresee the prospects of engineered fish. A regulatory program specifically targeted to the issues of genetically engineered fish and animals is urgently needed.[40]

Aqua Bounty Farms has wisely reduced the chance of a problem by promising either to grow its fish in recycled water facilities completely cut off from the ocean or to make sure that fish raised in ocean pens are sterile.[41] But it's not clear if these strategies will work perfectly, and the chances of a misstep will increase as more companies try to engineer fish.

---

research that should be carried out to monitor and reduce the impacts of agriculture on the environment.

Ideally, Waddell would like to see scientists agree to do a few side-by-side experiments comparing the performance of traditional and genetically engineered crops. If large test plots were planted and studied for 5 or 10 years, scientists could collect data to help resolve some of the questions about biotechnology.

But Waddell tries to think about food from more than just the scientist's perspective. Prior to obtaining his Ph.D. in ecology, he worked for 15 years in the food-service industry, where he learned what buyers must consider when they purchase staples at the commercial level and what chefs need to think about when they prepare and present food in ways that are attractive to local tastes and expectations. He also worked with apple and strawberry growers.

Although there were certainly significant differences among farmers, food buyers, and chefs, Waddell believes they all need to continually increase their knowledge in order to be successful in our fast-changing world. Scientists can help not only by expanding the knowledge base, but also by recommending adjustments that could reduce risks to the environment and public health. "By making adjustments to how we grow food," Waddell contends, "in the long run farming could be both more environmentally sustainable and more profitable."

SEPARATING THE WHEAT FROM THE CHAFF

The only reasonable way to proceed with genetic engineering is to have a strong government oversight system in place to ensure that only safe, useful products reach farmers' fields and grocery shelves. This will require a variety of improvements.

Both the perception and the reality has been that the U.S. government has been more concerned with promoting the biotechnology industry than closely regulating it. The USDA and U.S. trade officials have often acted as allies and advocates of the industry, frustrating not only environmental groups, but some farmers. Gary Goldberg, the head of the American Corn Growers Foundation, a small midwestern group, complains that "the USDA has been very unresponsive to any concerns, suggestions or ideas from farmers . . . They made a decision up front that they would support biotechnology at all costs, and that's what they're doing."[42]

The pro-biotech atmosphere at the Agriculture Department has been so strong that even the secretary of agriculture at the end of the Clinton administration, Dan Glickman, felt inhibited. "What I saw . . . ," he recalls, "was the attitude that the technology was good and that it was almost immoral to say that it wasn't good. . . . You felt you were almost an alien, disloyal, by trying to present an open-minded view on some of the issues being raised."[43]

Currently, three separate agencies, under the authority of three separate statutes, share responsibility for ensuring the safety of engineered foods, and none of them does an adequate job. A system that failed to foresee the taco shell fiascoes and allowed millions of acres of Bt crops to be grown before effective plans were in place to prevent the development of insect resistance is clearly inadequate. And because the technology is new, hard to understand, and unfamiliar, the public naturally has fears and concerns. Strong regulations can help the government and the biotech industry build public confidence and allay fears.

Genetically engineered foods are currently regulated by a patchwork system. The EPA puts plants with built-in pesticides, like Bt corn, through a formal approval process that is open to public scrutiny. But the FDA doesn't formally approve genetically engineered crops to ensure food safety. Rather, most of the safety review is handled by the biotechnology industry, instead of the government. Companies give the FDA test data to review on a confidential basis, until agency officials say "we have no further questions at this time." That secretive process hardly inspires public confidence. Instead, the FDA should actually determine the safety of crops using a mandatory approval process that is open to public examination and input.

In addition, all new genetically engineered crops should undergo a thorough environmental review. Such reviews should even be extended to some new nonbiotech crops. Herbicide-tolerant crops, for example, are entirely unregulated if they are developed without genetic modification.

To ensure that those genetically engineered crops that pose the greatest environmental risks receive especially close scrutiny from regulators, government scientists should work with impartial scientists from outside the government to develop clear standards for different categories of crops. They might, for example, establish a standard for plants that will be grown in close proximity to wild relatives, and another one for fish with traits that could increase their survivability in the wild. Standards should clearly delineate the specific types of genetically engineered crops that have already been proven safe, thereby requiring little additional oversight, and those that should be monitored carefully for years.

Scientists from outside the government should advise regulators when new, thorny, or controversial issues emerge. The EPA has moved in that direction by recently convening several panels of independent scientists on Bt corn and other issues. And, to avoid future taco-shell disasters, the agency will no longer allow food crops—either genetically engineered or conventional ones—to be grown for animal or industrial uses if they are not certified to be safe for human consumption.

In addition to careful scientific review and sound regulations, there needs to be stronger monitoring and enforcement mechanisms. The taco-shell case showed that lax field enforcement of guidelines set by the government can hurt consumer confidence.

CONSUMER INFORMATION

Today, with the new federal organic label that prohibits genetically engineered ingredients, consumers have an option that allows them to purchase biotech-free foods. But is that enough? Many opponents of biotechnology have advocated that all food containing genetically modified ingredients should carry a label. And indeed, numerous public opinion surveys have shown that consumers want information about whether the foods they buy are engineered. But coming up with an effective, fair, and economical way to provide this information is not simple.

At first glance, mandatory labeling of genetically engineered foods would seem to be the obvious answer. A poll conducted by the Center for Science in the Public Interest in April 2001 found that 62 to 70 percent of Americans want such foods to be labeled. However, they don't want labeling to be costly, and support for it drops to only 28 percent if it were to add $50 or more to a family's annual food costs.[44]

Devising a cost-effective and nondeceptive labeling scheme raises very difficult questions. For example, how should labeling treat soybean oil obtained from genetically engineered crops but which contains no modified DNA or proteins? Should beef be labeled if it was fattened on Bt corn, none of which remains in the meat? And, as the taco-shell case amply demonstrates, it is next to impossible to guarantee that small quantities of genetically modified foods won't get mixed in with conventional varieties somewhere along the way.

Some widely planted engineered foods, especially corn and soybeans, are minor ingredients in large numbers of prepared and packaged foods. If the government requires food with small amounts of genetically engineered ingredients to be labeled, food manufacturers might need to label almost everything (although, presumably, some threshold for accidental contamination would have to be permitted). The labels would quickly become meaningless if almost all the cans, boxes, and packages in the store said something vague like "may contain genetically engineered ingredients." On the other hand, requiring labeling only on foods where more than a small percentage (perhaps 3 to 5 percent) of the product has been genetically modified might leave consumers feeling deceived, since some foods without labels would still have genetically engineered content.[45]

An even bigger risk is that mandatory labeling would end up elimi-nating all genetically engineered ingredients from the food supply. In fact, this outcome is precisely what some labeling advocates hope for. They would like labels akin to a toxic warning. When mandatory label-ing was required in Europe, food processors reformulated their products to eliminate engineered ingredients, because they feared that some con-sumers would shun labeled products. Unless crafted carefully and ac-companied by proper consumer education, a mandatory labeling system might end up preventing consumers from having a choice between engi-neered and biotech-free foods, and society would lose the benefits of ge-netically engineered crops.

The FDA currently allows food manufacturers to voluntarily label their foods, but this approach does not give consumers the information or choice they desire. For fear of losing sales, no food company is cur-rently willing to label its products as containing genetically engineered ingredients—even if those ingredients lead to environmental benefits. Thus, the only foods labeled are ones that claim to be without those in-gredients. It turns out that not only are some of these claims untrue, but they are frequently expressed in a misleading or deceptive manner. Some manufacturers affix scary antibiotech labels onto their products in order to extract a premium price from consumers.

Of course, the food industry has brought much of this controversy upon itself. If food companies had been more open about their use of en-gineered ingredients—and even described the benefits on labels and in advertising—public suspicion might have been lessened and the contro-versy muted. Perhaps it is still not too late for food manufacturers to ad-vertise their use of ingredients made from engineered crops and explain the benefits and risks of such ingredients.

Labels aren't the only way for consumers to receive information about the foods they eat. For example, food companies could use web-sites and toll-free numbers to provide detailed information about the content of specific products. Most consumers, however, would find such strategies inconvenient.

No matter how consumers get information about whether the foods they eat contain genetically engineered ingredients, the information should be provided in a neutral way that does not imply a value judgment about the benefits or risks of biotechnology. The information should be truthful, avoid scary terms, avoid the appearance of a warning label, and not suggest that a product is superior simply because it does or does not contain genetically engineered ingredients. As biotech foods become more prevalent in our food supply, it is incumbent upon the government and industry to find a fair mechanism to get consumers the information they desire about the content of foods. Many consumers will not have confidence in genetically engineered foods if their existence is kept secret.

WHAT YOU CAN DO

Compared with the other topics discussed in this book, it is harder to take action on biotechnology at a grocery store or restaurant. If you are concerned about biotechnology for whatever reason, you can choose organic foods since they do not include genetically engineered ingredients. But given that the genetically modified foods on the market are safe and some even provide environmental benefits over traditionally grown crops, there is no need to worry about including them as part of your diet.

Some critics object to genetic engineering for ideological rather than scientific reasons. In Europe, for example, many people see biotechnology as part of an effort by big American companies to supplant local agricultural practices. In the United States, protesters at meetings of the World Trade Organization have used biotechnology to condemn global economic trends. As the British magazine *New Scientist* observes, for them "this controversy is really an emotional and political battle in a wider war against unfettered free trade, globalization and the power of multinationals."[46] While these issues are certainly important, they are distinct from the issue of whether genetically engineered foods are safe.

Agricultural biotechnology raises many other complex issues, such as the impact of biotechnology on small farmers; the failure of companies to develop improved fruit and vegetable crops; inadequate assistance to developing nations; increased corporate control over agriculture; the patenting of seeds; and other matters of great practical and philosophical importance. In terms of public policies, the United States certainly should be providing more aid to developing nations for agricultural improvements of all sorts, funding basic and applied research in this country to ensure that all developments are not controlled by industry, and ensuring that beneficial crops are developed that may not be of interest to the huge companies that dominate the industry.

Probably the most useful thing you can do is to follow news about the science and the politics of genetic engineering. Given how emotional the debate has become, it's not easy to find sound, objective information. The National Academy of Sciences (see www.nas.edu) is wrestling with the thorniest issues of genetic engineering in a sophisticated, serious way. Its reports are authoritative, although often technical. In Appendix B, we list some other useful information sources along with an indication of their point of view.

If you want to take action, you can focus on your role as a citizen rather than as a consumer. You can follow political developments and encourage your representatives in Congress, as well as officials in agencies like the EPA and the FDA, to support meaningful regulation of genetically engineered foods. To help the government and the country transcend the polarized debate over genetic engineering, people in the middle need to speak up. A few phone calls or letters could help make a difference.

CHAPTER SEVEN

MICROWAVE OVENS, SHADE-GROWN COFFEE, AND OTHER GOOD ENVIRONMENTAL CHOICES

We earlier looked at the environmental impacts of some of the major food groups, but other food choices also deserve scrutiny. This chapter looks at many of the food-related decisions concerned citizens ponder, including whether to wash dishes by hand or by machine, whether to eat at home or in a restaurant, and whether to choose locally grown food. We also cover which appliances and types of coffee are environmentally preferable.

NEARBY AND UNPROCESSED VERSUS DISTANT AND PROCESSED

Our earlier suggestion to buy locally grown food as a way to preserve local farmland and support good farms does not mean that the less distance the food travels to reach you the better it is for the environment. Moreover, processed foods can be sound environmental choices.

The vast majority of environmental damage related to food comes from growing the food rather than processing, packaging, or shipping it. To understand why, we need to remember that when we looked at the total share of consumers' environmental impacts coming from eating food, the greatest impacts were in the water-use and land-use categories. Virtually all the water use relates to cultivating and raising the food, not from other stages in the production process.

In terms of land use, although processing, packaging, and transportation have impacts (for example, trees are used to make cardboard for food packages and food distribution facilities take up land), the impacts of raising the food are many times greater.

The water-pollution impacts of food choices are also quite serious, but here, too, most are caused by food cultivation—namely animal waste and the use of pesticides and chemical fertilizers. Processing, packaging, and shipping play significant roles only for air pollution and global warming, a consequence primarily of energy use. Yet even for air pollution, the food-raising stage remains more significant, since farm machinery with its poor pollution controls produces considerable air pollution, as does the manufacture and use of pesticides, fertilizers, and other inputs into the farming process.

When it comes to global warming, processing and shipping are more important factors than raising the food. The impacts are roughly proportional to the use of fossil fuels for energy (although for a few foods, other factors such as methane emissions from cattle's belching play an important role). But keep in mind that food overall causes only 12 percent of consumers' total contribution to global warming; driving cars and using energy in homes are *much* greater contributors to global warming.

Figure 9 takes the broad category of "fruits, vegetables, and grains" and shows where the environmental impacts of the cultivation stage of the food-production process exceeds the combined impacts of food processing, packaging, and shipping. A more detailed table, which breaks down the impacts of food processing versus packaging versus shipping, is available in the endnotes.[1]

There are circumstances in which food processing and packaging can actually be good for the environment. In some cases they eliminate food spoilage, cut down on food waste, or reduce the weight and bulk of shipping the food to consumers. To take an extreme example, it's better for the environment—though not for taste or nutrition—to produce orange juice near the orange grove than to ship whole oranges to stores and ask consumers to squeeze their own. Fewer oranges go bad and have to be thrown out; fewer trucks and less energy are needed to ship the juice. As another example, bruised apples or tomatoes that consumers would reject if they were displayed in the supermarket are turned into applesauce or tomato sauce. In general, food processing is a time-honored way to use food that would otherwise go to waste.

Of course, some food products are overpackaged, and manufacturers should be encouraged to eliminate unnecessary packaging. In addition, many processed foods contain high levels of salts, sugars, and fats, there-

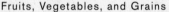

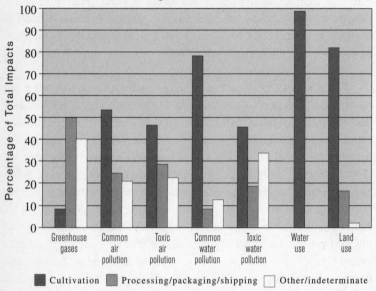

FIGURE 9
WHERE THE IMPACTS OCCUR

Fruits, Vegetables, and Grains

■ Cultivation   ■ Processing/packaging/shipping   □ Other/indeterminate

fore making them nutritionally inferior. But don't reject all packaged and processed foods for environmental reasons.

Similarly, don't make the geographic origins of food your overriding concern. It's not going to matter much if potatoes come from 500 or 1,500 miles away. And don't choose conventional apples from across the state over organic apples from across the country. But if you can find local, *sustainably grown* food, you've done the best of all.

COFFEE THAT MAKES A DIFFERENCE

If it would save the habitats of America's songbirds, reduce pesticide pollution, and help lift beleaguered coffee workers out of crushing poverty, would you pay four cents extra for your next cup of coffee?

That's all it would take to help reverse some disastrous environmental and economic trends.

Traditional coffee growing is an unusually environmentally friendly form of agriculture. Coffee plants love shade, so farmers in Latin America, the world's major coffee-producing region, used to plant them under a canopy of trees. The trees not only protected the coffee plants from too much sun or rain, but they cut down on weeds and provided mulch, reducing the need for chemical fertilizers.[2]

By mixing many varieties of trees, often 25 or more different types on a single plantation, coffee farmers unintentionally created the next-best habitat to a wild forest for birds, insects, and other wildlife. Many songbirds that summer in the United States spend their winters on coffee farms in northern Latin America. As the region's forests have been cut down, the coffee plantations have become ever more important. In El Salvador, for example, more than half the remaining forested areas are coffee plantations.[3]

Unfortunately, starting in the 1970s, a different type of coffee farming began to take root. Governments and farmers worried that the arrival in Latin America of coffee leaf rust, a potentially devastating plant disease, threatened the region's continued ability to produce coffee. As a solution to this threat, the U.S. Agency for International Development promoted a modernized style of coffee production that replaced traditional varieties of coffee with newer ones while also helping farmers to increase production. The new varieties could be grown in the sun, but required chemical fertilizers and pesticides. The shade trees started to come down, while water pollution and worker illnesses from pesticides went up. When scientists in Colombia and Mexico counted how many birds remained, they found 94 to 97 percent fewer bird species where coffee is grown in the sun rather than the shade.[4]

During the 1990s, additional new strains of coffee and more intensive farming methods created an ever larger supply of coffee. Additional countries, most notably Vietnam, which quickly became the world's second-largest producer, entered the market. Despite the spread of coffee bars and the premium-coffee craze in the United States and Europe, the supply of coffee worldwide grew twice as fast as consumption did. As a result, between 1998 and 2001, prices crashed from $1.34 per pound to under

$0.50. At these low prices, many farmers can't even recoup their production costs.[5]

Consumers haven't seen much savings from the coffee glut, but Nestlé and other big coffee-processing companies, along with retailers like Starbucks, have reaped a windfall. Over the past 10 years, the total amount of money the world's consumers pay for coffee has increased from $30 billion to $50 billion, but the amount going to coffee producers actually fell by $4 billion, and now represents only 16 percent of the total, compared with 40 percent at the beginning of the 10-year period.[6]

Many coffee farmers have been thrown into ever-deeper poverty. As one small-scale Tanzanian farmer laments, "Years back, when coffee prices were good, we could afford to send our children to school. Now we are taking our children out of school because we cannot afford the fees. How can we send our children to school when we cannot afford to feed them well?" A Nicaraguan mother who skips eating on some days exclaims that "the children cry from hunger. There is no work. The coffee growers cannot get money to pay us."[7]

Because 20 million households around the world are involved in coffee farming, the current situation represents a serious human crisis that governments and international agencies need to address. But various private organizations have already been working on one solution—reinvigorating traditional, small-scale, environmentally friendly coffee farming. In some cases, they are doing this for primarily environmental reasons; in other cases, to ensure that coffee farmers receive a living wage. The Smithsonian Migratory Bird Center labels some sustainably grown shade coffee with a Bird Friendly logo. The Rainforest Alliance has slightly different criteria for its Eco-OK coffee. TransFair USA promotes Fair Trade Certified coffee, which guarantees that farmers receive a fair price, about 2.5 times higher than today's current depressed price. There's also organic coffee, which meets the same standards that organic farmers in the United States must achieve, but may not be shade grown, although most is.

In the long run, it would be better for consumers if all the groups interested in sustainable coffee would agree on a single set of criteria and a single logo. Today, however, don't worry too much about which logo or label is best, since all the labels we just mentioned tend to reward environmentally sound farmers with premium prices. There is considerable overlap among them. For example, 85 percent of Fair Trade Certified coffee is shade grown and either certified organic or produced using similar methods. Although they cost more, it's not a lot given what you are accomplishing. If you have to pay an extra $2 per pound for coffee, this works out to only about $0.04 extra for every cup you brew.

Because coffee is our nation's largest food import, Americans have a responsibility to take action. Our consumer purchases can make a big difference. Your morning cup of coffee will taste better if you know you are helping seriously underpaid farmers and preserving crucial animal habitats. You'll be assisting people like Ramirez Lopez, a Guatemalan Fair Trade farmer, who recently said, "Not only do I not walk in bare feet anymore, I am a much better farmer."[8]

EATING OUT OR EATING IN?

In terms of the environment, it doesn't make a tremendous difference whether you eat at home or in a restaurant, as long as you eat the same environmentally sound foods. Of course, in specific cases there could be an advantage to eating in or eating out. For example, it would be a sound choice to eat in a restaurant that serves organic vegetables or sustainably caught fish. You might do better to eat at home if you know you are unusually efficient in your use of energy and water for cooking and cleaning up. But most differences in eating location are hard to assess with any accuracy. So, in general, give your greatest attention to what you eat rather than where you eat.

Nevertheless, there are two ways in which restaurant dining can be problematic. First, because driving to the restaurant causes considerable air pollution and global warming,[9] you can minimize these impacts by choosing restaurants close to home, or combine eating with other trips. Of course, almost everyone spontaneously goes out on occasion, but as a general rule it's good to limit the number of such trips and to develop an overall plan for reducing the amount of driving you do.

Second, many restaurants revel in (or perhaps we should say wallow in) excess by consciously serving patrons ludicrously large portions. If you get twice as much food as you need, and half of it ends up in the trash, the environmental impact of your meal is roughly twice as large as it should be. (Of course, the solution is not to eat more than you want to so that you leave the restaurant feeling bloated.) Plan to eat only half your meal, and take the leftovers home to eat later.

PREPARING, STORING, SERVING, AND CLEANING UP FOOD

Appliances

When it comes to the environmental impacts of preparing, storing, serving, and cleaning up food, your appliances deserve the most attention. The energy required to run appliances produces air pollution and contributes to global warming. Some appliances, like gas stoves, run on natural gas, but most are electric. Although electricity seems clean and nonpolluting when it's used in the home, most of it is generated by burn-

---

GOOD FISH ON THE MENU

For Steve Johnson, implementing his environmental principles requires a discerning and critical eye. As the chef and co-owner of the Blue Room, an eclectic contemporary American restaurant in Cambridge, Massachusetts, he also needs to have a juggler's talents in order to respond to his customers' preferences while trying to serve local food that is raised or caught using sustainable methods.

As a founding member of the Boston chapter of the Chef's Collaborative, a network of chefs and restaurateurs who promote sustainable cuisine, Johnson supports local producers whenever possible. During the short New England growing season, he purchases produce from a local organic farmer and says his patrons can taste the difference. But the challenges are greater when it comes to seafood.

Although a wide variety of fish species that provide delicious menu options year-round swim in the waters off Boston, suppliers cannot always guarantee that their fish was caught locally. Johnson therefore tries to know the local fishers and supports those who use sustainable fishing practices. As an important part of his work with the Chef's Collaborative, he helps local producers overcome the obstacles to bringing their products to the local market. By helping them deal with the challenges created by the consolidation of the food industry, he can also offer the freshest, highest-quality food to his customers.

ing polluting fossil fuels, especially coal. By taking steps to use less energy, you will not only cut down on pollution, but save money on your utility bills.

It's helpful to train yourself to avoid unnecessary appliance use by such things as running the dishwasher only when it's full and not leaving the refrigerator door open for long periods of time. But by far the most important thing to do is to buy efficient, low-polluting appliances in the first place. By buying the most efficient models, you will use up to 40 percent less electricity than if you buy the least efficient one of the same size, thereby causing 40 percent less of the air pollution and greenhouse gases associated with electrical generation. At-home conservation measures, such as regularly vacuuming refrigerator coils, can't achieve anywhere near this large a reduction. This doesn't mean that you should ignore such everyday actions, but the moment at which you produce

Some of the best seasonal seafood choices from an environmental perspective are unfamiliar to most restaurant goers, but Johnson tries to feature them on the Blue Room's menu. By offering these unusual fish, he increases awareness of local seafood while adding variety and interest to his menu. Many of his customers know and agree with this philosophy; others just know that they enjoy the food. Either way, Johnson influences his customers with his menu selections. He feels fortunate that the abundance of fish varieties in New England affords him the flexibility to offer many popular seafood choices to his customers. His task would be more difficult in some other parts of the country.

Johnson acknowledges that he sometimes must balance his personal ideology against customer demand for seafood like tuna that is not caught locally. Recognizing this, he devotes his greatest energy to where he can make the greatest impact—improving awareness in the food industry by developing relationships with trusted suppliers and spreading the message to other local chefs. It's a win-win situation because his suppliers understand and strive to meet his high standards while his customers enjoy safe, high-quality food. When he serves smelts or other underutilized local fish, and they swim off the menu with rave reviews, he knows he has done his job on many levels.

the largest effect—either positive or negative—is when you buy a new model.

Luckily, the U.S. Environmental Protection Agency and the U.S. Department of Energy now make it easy for you to make good appliance choices by awarding an Energy Star logo to the more efficient refrigerators and dishwashers. You can get a list of the Energy Star–rated appliances by going to the Energy Star website: www.energystar.gov. There is also a useful list of the top-rated appliances at the website of the American Council for an Energy-Efficient Economy (www.aceee.org), derived from its book *Consumer Guide to Home Energy Savings.* And *Consumer Reports* periodically publishes useful articles.

Refrigerators

When you think about the environmental impacts of your appliances, start with your refrigerator, since it's the biggest energy hog in your kitchen. This makes sense, given that it's a big machine that's in use 24 hours a day, 365 days a year.

Some people hang on to a 25-year-old refrigerator thinking that they are being frugal and good for the environment, but in reality they are causing considerable unnecessary environmental damage. Over the past 25 years, refrigerators have become three times more efficient. That means that old ones cause three times more polluting coal to be burned than is necessary. They also cost an additional $50, $75, or even more to run each year than an efficient new model.

Because of the considerable savings on electricity costs, a new refrigerator may ultimately pay for itself. Even if you purchased one as recently as 10 years ago, you may consider replacing it.

When looking for a new refrigerator, try not to get one larger (and therefore more energy-consuming) than you really need. On the other hand, if you need extra storage, rather than move your old refrigerator to the basement for that purpose, purchase a larger refrigerator, since a single big one will use much less electricity than two smaller ones or a refrigerator and a separate, freestanding freezer.

In general, top or bottom freezer models are more efficient than side-by-side ones, and extra gizmos like water dispensers add to the electricity use. But to get the best model for your needs, look first for the Energy

Star logo and then compare the estimated electricity costs on the labels of the various Energy Star models you like.

Dishwashing

Some people avoid using dishwashing machines to avoid the environmental damage associated with using electricity to run the machine. Indeed, a very careful hand washer can probably clean dishes while using less water and energy than a machine. But for the average person who tends to be less zealous when washing dishes by hand, a machine compares favorably with hand washing, because the machine is designed to use water—and especially hot water—efficiently. It is also more sanitary, as it can use water hot enough to scald a human.

For an automatic dishwasher to be a good choice environmentally, choose an efficient model. You should also avoid washing the dishes twice—once by hand and once by machine. Many people, perhaps remembering long-ago lessons from their mothers or the poor quality of early dishwashing machines, rinse the dishes before placing them in the dishwasher. This is a waste of time, water, and energy! Unless the dishes have materials on them that require scrubbing—melted cheese and the like—a good modern dishwashing machine will get them clean without any prerinsing by hand.

Electric Versus Gas Ranges

In general, gas stoves use less energy than electric models. Also, gas stoves do a better job of cooking, so it's not surprising that professional cooks prefer gas to electric. If you use the oven frequently, make sure to get a self-cleaning model, since it will be better insulated and therefore more energy efficient.

Microwave Ovens

If you have a choice of cooking appliance, use a microwave. It uses much less energy than a conventional oven. It throws off less heat into your kitchen, which keeps your kitchen cooler and saves on summer air-conditioning costs. The American Council for an Energy-Efficient

Economy has estimated the relative costs and energy use of different methods for cooking the same casserole. What would take an hour in a 350-degree electric oven takes only one-quarter of that, or 15 minutes, in a microwave. The difference in energy used and expense is even greater—2.00 kilowatt hours and 16 cents versus 0.36 kilowatt hours and 3 cents. Although Crock-Pots, toaster ovens, frying pans, gas ovens, and electric convection ovens are all more efficient than a large electric oven, a microwave is two to nearly four times better than any of these alternatives.[10]

There are some minor risks from microwaves, primarily from ingesting contaminants from plastic containers or wraps that come in contact with oily foods. To reduce these risks, microwave food on glass or ceramic plates and bowls or on plastic ones marked microwave-safe.

Outdoor Grills

Traditional charcoal and wood grills produce some of the best-tasting food, but they also emit much more air pollution than gas and electric grills. An occasional use or two won't really matter, but if you grill frequently you should try to stay away from charcoal and wood. Even if you sacrifice a little of that smoky barbecue taste, you can take solace from the fact that gas and electric grills are much easier and more convenient to use.

Disposable Cups, Plates, Plastic Utensils, Paper Towels, and Paper Napkins

The throwaway drink cup has become a powerful symbol of America's wasteful, polluting society. Nevertheless, it is not a major sin against the environment to use an occasional paper or plastic cup. These lightweight products require relatively little energy to make and take up little space in landfills. Of course, you don't want to be wasteful, but a few dozen disposable cups a year will have relatively little environmental impact.

Similarly, when it comes to paper plates, plastic utensils, and paper products, quantity is key. Although it is, of course, best to avoid wasting materials, you should consider how much waste is involved. If you ate every meal using onetime-use plastic utensils and paper plates, it would not only be unnecessarily wasteful but would cost more money than washing dishes. (However, we must remember that dishwashing also requires resources—water for cleaning and fossil fuels or some other energy source for heating the water.)

An occasional picnic or purchase from a take-out restaurant has little environmental impact and is not a cause for concern. If you keep in mind the 20 tons of animal waste that the average household indirectly generates by its consumption of meat and dairy, it puts the disposable-products issue into perspective.

If you are going to use disposable products, look for ones made from recycled materials. Several companies make paper towels and napkins made from recycled paper; other recycled disposable products are harder to find.

Styrofoam Cups and Spray Cans

Here, too, quantity is key, and you should feel fine about using these items in nonwasteful amounts. Many people continue to avoid these products because back in the 1970s they used chlorofluorocarbons that depleted the ozone layer. In response to consumer pressure and government regulations, manufacturers changed production methods, which relieves the guilt about using polystyrene (Styrofoam) cups or aerosol cans for spraying cooking oil, whipped cream, and other food products.

Paper or Plastic?

Finally, what should you answer when the grocery store clerk asks, "Paper or plastic?" Frankly, that is really not an important environmental decision and you should pick whichever type of bag you find most convenient.

It is far from obvious which of the two bags is even marginally better for the environment. In the 1980s, many supermarkets tried to shift from paper bags to plastic, since the plastic (polyethylene) sacks were less expensive. Because so many customers complained—partly because the plastic bags were flimsier, but also because they thought plastic was a less environment-friendly material than paper—most food stores ultimately gave customers a choice between the two bag types.

Not surprisingly, the plastic manufacturers were unwilling to concede that their product was environmentally inferior, and they funded studies to show its advantages. In a thorough analysis of the two types of grocery bags, the consulting firm Franklin Associates concluded that the manufacture of plastic sacks actually produced considerably less air pollution, waterborne wastes, and industrial solid waste than paper. Because plastic bags were much lighter, they also took up less space in landfills. (In the airless conditions of the typical landfill, paper, which is biodegradable, tends not to degrade.) The researchers found that plastic sacks continued to have those advantages even when they assumed that grocery store clerks packed less in each bag, thereby requiring 1.5 or 2 times as many bags to pack the same quantity of groceries as with paper.[11]

It was less clear which type of sack was preferable in terms of energy use. Plastic bags required less overall energy to manufacture when the researchers assumed the grocery store baggers used 1.5 times the number of paper bags, but about the same amount of energy when twice as many plastic bags were used, with relatively high recycling rates.[12] Moreover, much of the energy for making paper bags came from a renewable energy source—wood.

On balance, plastic sacks seem to have come out as the environmentally better choice. However, to even things out, we should keep in mind that paper grocery bags are reused more frequently, since many home kitchen trash containers are designed with paper grocery sacks in mind. Of course, bringing your own cloth bags or asking store clerks to give you your purchases without bags will reduce the waste and do away with the dilemma. But no matter what you do, it's not all that big a deal.

CHAPTER EIGHT

BUILDING
THE SAFEST FOOD SUPPLY:
A MENU OF ACTIONS TO IMPROVE
YOUR COMMUNITY AND
INFLUENCE THE GOVERNMENT

"America has the safest food supply in the world." This mantra is repeated over and over by the food industry and the government. It is the "don't worry, be happy" answer to many of the food-safety and environmental issues raised by consumer and environmental organizations.

Although our food supply is generally quite safe and certainly bountiful, there is little evidence that the U.S. food system is safer than all others. Our country certainly doesn't hold a monopoly on strong food-safety and environmental standards. In fact, countries in Europe, as well as Canada, have stronger standards for certain food issues. Sweden, for example, eradicated chicken flocks infected with *Salmonella* 20 years ago, which has helped to reduce human *Salmonella* infections. Canada inspects seafood plants much more frequently than the United States does. The European Union has banned the use in animal production of most of the antibiotics that are essential in treating human illnesses. In other areas, however, the United States is stronger. For example, the Food and Drug Administration (FDA) banned the production of some types of cheese from unpasteurized milk in order to reduce deaths and illnesses from *Listeria*. In addition, a ban on certain cattle and beef products by the U.S. Department of Agriculture (USDA) beginning in 1989 has so far prevented mad cow disease from spreading to the United States.

While consumers can have a huge impact on food safety and the environment by adjusting their purchasing behavior, they can't very easily monitor the overall safety of the food supply. Instead, consumers must rely on government agencies like the FDA, the USDA, and the Environmental Protection Agency (EPA) to set food-safety standards and assure that farmers and food processors are complying. But these agencies won't be as vigilant as necessary unless they and our elected representatives truly believe that the public places a high priority on food safety and is watching to make sure that they follow through.

The dedicated efforts of citizen activists, like Nancy Donley, and committed Washington insiders, like Carol Tucker Foreman, have precipitated significant improvements in the safety of the American food supply. Although our society certainly needs more such people, you don't have to become a full-time activist or lobbyist to have an impact on the government's policies. Often just a few hours of your time can make a difference in how a local agency, like your community's health department, acts or how one of your elected representatives votes on food-safety legislation. It won't be easy to achieve positive results, but it is always worth putting in a little time and creative energy to try to ensure that America's food is the safest in the world.

The methods you can use to influence your community and various governments may not seem novel, but they have repeatedly been proven to work: keeping informed about what governments and your elected representatives are doing about food safety; voting and working for candidates who will make food safety a priority; contacting your elected officials to express your views; writing letters to newspapers to influence public understanding of food safety; helping organizations that are working for sound government policies; and talking to and cooperating with people in your community who affect the safety of the local food supply.

Here is a menu of actions you could take to improve the food system in your community and in the country as a whole. Although there are certainly other, equally meaningful steps you could take to ensure the safety of the food supply, the five local and six national actions outlined in the following pages are not only highly desirable, but need the help of people like you if they are going to happen.

ACT LOCALLY

EFFECTIVE LOCAL ACTIONS

1. Reduce contaminants in your drinking water.
2. Strengthen local restaurant inspections.
3. Improve school food.
4. Assist family farms and expand farmers' markets.
5. Get better foods into local stores and restaurants.

1. Reduce Contaminants in Your Drinking Water

Drinking water can harbor both chemical and microbiological hazards. Luckily, your access to information about drinking water is better than ever before. Every year, the local suppliers of drinking water are required to send out consumer-confidence reports, which provide information about the safety of water in your area. These reports are frequently distributed by mail and include information on where the water comes from, results of monitoring for contamination, and information on health concerns. If you haven't received this report in the last year, call your state and local water utility. The EPA also runs a hotline (800-426-4791) to help you get information on whom to contact.

Approximately 55,000 community water systems are required by law to test for more than 80 contaminants. In 1998, about 6 percent of those systems failed one or more health standards for drinking water. When a safety standard for drinking water is exceeded, the community water system must alert the public to the problem. These notices give consumers an effective way to monitor the performance of the water authority in their area.

If a contaminant poses an immediate health hazard, suppliers must notify their customers within 24 hours. These announcements will typically be made through the local media and may include instructions to boil water. Other violations will likely be included with water bills.

You can take the following steps to monitor and improve the safety of your drinking water.

- Call your state and local water authority and check to see that monitoring and reporting requirements are being met. In most places, tests for bacteria and viruses are conducted monthly. Lead and copper are checked annually. These tests are critical to ensure that problems are discovered and corrected.

- Enlist an organization or local media to help you check the information on the consumer-confidence reports. A survey of California water utilities conducted in 2001 by several environmental groups found tremendous variability in these reports, with smaller utilities failing most frequently to distribute complete water-quality information to their customers. Many utilities failed to disclose the sources for the contaminants in the water and did not publicize meetings. In addition, the reports are frequently available only in English, which is a disservice to consumers who do not speak English.

- Help protect the source waters. With drinking water, as with most other things, preventing a problem is better than curing it. Check with your local water supplier to see if there is a source water protection program. Source water protection is an even greater concern since the September 11, 2001, terrorist attacks. If you live nearby, enlist your friends and neighbors to ensure that the land closest to the water intake is used appropriately to minimize the likelihood of contamination of the water and report any suspicious activity to authorities.

- Educate small polluters, including your friends and neighbors, on safe disposal practices. Don't dump household chemicals and solvents

---

CITIZEN ACTION MAKES THE DIFFERENCE

The cleanup of an Acton, Massachusetts, industrial site is still not complete 23 years after local citizens began protesting that it was contaminating the local drinking water. Yet Charlotte Sagoff and Robert Eisengrein, two leaders of the citizens group, believe that their experience shows that citizen action can be effective and not that difficult.

Back in the 1970s, the town of Acton needed to increase its water supply. But when three test wells were drilled near the site of a W. R. Grace & Company facility, the water had a strong chemical odor. In retrospect, this was not surprising, since the company was dumping chemical waste into unlined lagoons, from which it could easily seep into the ground. The evidence of groundwater contamination caused some local residents to question the safety of two nearby existing wells that were already supplying much of the town's water.

The problem was addressed in stages. First, the two wells were closed. Second, W. R. Grace was found responsible for causing the water contamination. The company was then held to a commitment to clean up its site. Although various local, state, and federal agencies all played important roles, the small band of citizen activists made a crucial difference. Through their organization, Acton Citizens for Environmental Safety (ACES), led by Sagoff, they kept the problem in

down the drain. Make sure that household hazardous wastes, such as paint and thinners, pesticides, and used oil, are collected regularly.

- Participate in decisions about which projects your state will fund to improve the safety and quality of the drinking water. States and local authorities must consult with the public on these key decisions.

- Encourage a local environmental group to file a citizen suit under the federal Safe Drinking Water Act if your state or local water authority is not complying with the law. You have the right to enforce it!

- If you rely on a private well, get it tested at least once a year for nitrate and coliform bacteria. These tests will cost about $10 to $20. Check for chemicals and other hazards whenever you suspect

---

the public eye and made it impossible for the company or the town to sweep it under the rug.

Government and company officials knew that ACES would always have a representative at any public meeting, so they needed to be prepared with answers. To ensure news coverage of the meetings, Sagoff would alert the local newspaper that ACES was going to be there asking tough questions. Letters in the newspaper from the group's members also provided valuable publicity.

As a recipe for effective citizen action to solve a problem, Sagoff believes that having an organization is key, since it gives activists an official status. But the group doesn't need to be large. To get started, Sagoff recommends "inviting a few concerned neighbors over to your house for tea. Then ask them to invite a few of the people they know to join."

Eisengrein has represented ACES in countless meetings with the Grace company and the EPA over the past decade. "Citizens have more power than they realize," he observes. "Just looking over the shoulders of offending companies and public officials keeps pressure on them and encourages them to do a better job. You don't need a Ph.D. to ask the obvious questions and insist they be answered in public meetings."

Acton now has some of the safest water in the state, and with ACES' help, it's protected for the future.

a problem. Consult local resources, such as the extension service or your university, on how to correct contamination problems that you find in your well water.

2. Strengthen Local Restaurant Inspections

Americans eat more and more meals away from home. While we can control conditions in our own kitchens, it is much harder to manage food-safety risks, as well as dietary choices, away from home. Local and state governments are the ones responsible for inspecting local restaurants.

Several years ago, the Center for Science in the Public Interest (CSPI) surveyed nearly 50 state and local agencies that conduct restaurant inspections. The findings were quite troubling. Even though the fed-

---

A SALAD BAR GOES TO SCHOOL

When Pat Malloy agreed to accompany her husband to a public forum on organic farming and community agriculture, she didn't realize that it would lead to a major overhaul of the food offerings in her children's elementary school in Ventura, California. But she became excited when she heard a speaker from Occidental College's Community Food Security Program describe how a Santa Monica school had set up a salad bar in the school cafeteria, serving food from the local farmers' market. Malloy, a former health education teacher, had already been interested in getting more fresh foods included in the lunches at her children's school and decided that a farmers' market salad bar would be a great way to accomplish this.

Malloy convinced the Juanamaria Elementary School food service director and a school board member to support the salad bar concept. Even though school administrators strongly supported the project, they were skeptical that it would actually get students to eat more vegetables. But Malloy and other parents were determined to give it a try. Her husband and another parent secured several grants to get things started.

Now that the salad bar has become a reality, it has become the most popular lunch offering at the school. On some days 300 of the 500 children at the school choose the salad bar over the school lunch program's hot-meal option.

eral government has recommended that states and localities adopt specific Food Code standards for the inspection of restaurants, such standards weren't being used by a large number of the agencies surveyed. In fact, important food-safety measures, such as cooking temperatures for hamburgers and eggs, were not being adequately enforced. Here's how to check up on local enforcement of safety standards in the restaurants near you.

- Ask your city or county health department for a copy of your local restaurant inspection standards and compare it with the federal Food Code, available through the Food and Drug Administration at www.cfsan.fda.gov/~dms/foodcode.html. Document the differences, and give this information to a local reporter. Lobby your local and state health departments to amend your local code to ensure that it is at least as strong as the federal standards.

What produced this great success was careful planning and Malloy's commitment to linking the lunch program to nutrition education. Before the salad bar was installed, Malloy spent time promoting it to students, teachers, and school administrators. Now that the salad bar is up and running, she goes to the farmers' market every week and brings back a different or new vegetable to the classrooms. She talks to the students about the vegetables and brings in samples for them, giving meaning and familiarity to the food.

At the salad bar, parent volunteers encourage the children to make selections that fit with the recommendations of the National School Lunch Program. The volunteers include all of the food groups on the salad bar, and they help keep down fat and sodium intake by monitoring salad dressing portions.

The students have caught Malloy's contagious enthusiasm for the salad bar project. Because they have been given responsibility for choosing their own selections with only modest guidance, they have a sense of ownership in the project.

With the salad bar well established, Malloy and the other parent volunteers are now working to start a school garden program. Malloy also has other ideas for improving students' health and understanding of food, including increasing physical activity and school food composting.

- Lobby to get restaurant inspection results posted in the restaurants. This has already been done in a number of places, with great success. For example, after Los Angeles required restaurants to post their inspection "grade" in the window, the percentage of restaurants earning an A jumped from 40 percent to 75 percent in just two years.

- Restaurant inspection reports should be easily available to the public in the newspaper, through a well-publicized phone number, and over the Internet. This has already been done in many areas of the country, including Alaska, Florida, North Carolina, and southern California. If your area hasn't adopted these methods to provide quick public access to information yet, your actions could change that.

- If you can't get help from the agency in charge of inspecting restaurants, work with the local media to get an investigation of restaurant inspection reports. While a good investigative report can take months of work, the media exposure is likely to result in quick and positive changes in the safety practices of local restaurants. Media reports will also create interest among local politicians to ensure the public availability of inspection reports.

- Support state legislation to get restaurants to disclose nutritional information on their menu boards and menus. Given the growth in restaurant and restaurant-prepared meals, prominent disclosure of calories and other nutritional information would help consumers make better dietary choices.

3. Improve School Food

One of the best places to make a change that could have a lasting impact is in your local elementary schools. Children eat one or two meals a day at school, and this means that food safety and nutrition may be nearly as important as the education offered there. Schools have slipped into a number of bad habits over the years. They are given or purchase food from the federal government that can be high in fat. The school cooks must then try to incorporate this food into healthy meals. In addition, soft-drink companies have used schools as marketing opportunities. These companies have funded athletic teams and other activities in exchange for having vending machines in the school.

The next time you are in your child's school, swing by the kitchen and talk to the staff there. The person who is in charge of the kitchen will probably enjoy the recognition that his or her job is an important one. Make each visit a friendly one, and try to learn about how the kitchen functions. The job of providing healthy, nutritious food to hundreds of children every day is a challenging one, especially as federal subsidies for the food programs have declined and as kids have grown accustomed to eating junk food outside of school.

Here are some ideas for improving food safety and nutrition in your local schools.

- Ask how purchasing decisions for meat and other foods are made. Is the meat tested for harmful bacteria, like *Salmonella*? Find out from the local health department the date of the last inspection of the school kitchen and cafeteria. Ask to see the report.

- Ask to see a nutrition analysis of the meals being offered. Are the schools serving full-fat or low-fat milk? Is the pizza made with a whole-wheat crust and low-fat cheese? Remember, nutritious food may be more expensive, so you might have to lobby to get more funding for the school lunch program in your state.

- Tell the principal you want him or her to keep junk food out of your child's school. If soda and candy vending machines are already there, raise the issue in the PTA meetings. Start a campaign to get the junk food out of the schools and form alliances with local dentists and nutritionists. Having a diverse group support your efforts will be most effective. Look for support on the school board.

4. Assist Family Farms and Expand Farmers' Markets

Getting to know your local farmers and food producers is a wonderful antidote to many of the problems with modern agriculture. Many farmers do not make an adequate living, and frequently much of the profit goes to middlemen.

- Lobby your mayor and city, town, or county council for more space for farmers' markets in your community. Eastern Market in Washington, D.C., and Union Square in New York City are excellent examples of how urban spaces can be adapted to attract farmers and other sellers. More spaces like this will connect farmers to consumers.

- Join a local Community Supported Agriculture (CSA) cooperative. If you can't join one, create one. CSA members pledge to support the operating costs for a single farm or farming cooperative for a season and then share the harvest, frequently delivered fresh from the farm. CSA co-ops can be set up in offices, apartment buildings, and even neighborhoods.

5. Get Better Foods into Local Stores and Restaurants

Through buying decisions, you let food store managers know which foods you like. But there are additional ways to provide food stores and restaurants with feedback, although few people take advantage of them. These businesses are interested in hearing from their customers. Here are a few things you might do.

- When your food store has especially good or varied organic produce in stock, be sure to buy some and let the manager know that you noticed and appreciate the store's efforts.

- If the store carries organic or other sustainably raised meats, choose them rather than conventional ones. If they aren't there, request that the store stock organic meat and produce.

- Ask your food store to let shoppers know when a particular display of fruits or vegetables comes from local farms.

- If a restaurant has obvious food-safety problems, such as buffet food that is lukewarm when it should be hot, report these conditions to the local public health department.

- If a restaurant has taken steps to use local produce, organic foods, or sustainably caught fish, let the staff know that you appreciate their efforts.

MAKE YOUR VOICE HEARD IN WASHINGTON

National food-policy debates are frequently dominated by big food companies and trade associations who want to minimize regulations regardless of the health consequences. It is essential that members of Congress and officials in government agencies hear other voices as well. Although working to promote change at the national level can seem challenging, like David against Goliath, persistent citizens can make a difference. Here are some suggestions for activities that could have big consequences.

IMPORTANT NATIONAL ACTIONS

1. Reduce the use of antibiotics in agriculture.

2. Clean up meat, poultry, and seafood.

3. Reduce animal waste and recycle it safely.

4. Fully implement the Food Quality Protection Act.

5. Strengthen the regulation of genetically modified foods.

6. Create a single food-safety agency.

---

1. Reduce the Use of Antibiotics in Agriculture

Most of the antibiotics produced in the United States are used in agricultural production. While some are used to treat diseases in animals, most are used to fatten animals faster. Such nontherapeutic use of antibiotics greatly increases the likelihood that bacteria will develop resistance.

Feeding low levels of antibiotics to healthy animals allows for more intensive farming of animals and crowded conditions that promote diseases. The benefits to the growers are not worth the risk to public health. For example, antibiotic-resistant bacteria on food can cause severe food poisoning that is hard to treat.

Numerous health organizations, including the World Health Organization and the American Medical Association, have called for a ban on the subtherapeutic use of medically important antibiotics in animal agriculture. Here's what you could do.

• Write to your senators and congressperson to urge them to support legislation that would ban all nontherapeutic uses of antimicrobial agents that are used in human medicine or are closely related to ones used in human medicine.

- Write to the EPA (410 M Street, S.W., Washington, D.C. 20460) to urge that the agency ban the use of antibiotics as pesticides. Antibiotics are applied to fruit trees each year to treat bacterial infections. This practice may create new strains of resistant bacteria and creates the opportunity to transfer these resistant genes to human pathogens.

- Ask your grocer to stock meat and poultry raised without antibiotics.

2. Clean Up Meat, Poultry, and Seafood

Although the federal government has implemented new systems to improve the safety of these foods, much remains to be done. The FDA has not required safety testing of seafood products, and industry compliance remains low. While the federal meat and poultry inspection system has stronger testing requirements, the meat and poultry industries try to weaken these safeguards. And both the USDA and the FDA lack such basic enforcement tools as mandatory recall of unsafe food and civil fines for repeat violators. Here are some steps you can take.

- Write to your congressperson and senators, urging them to support legislation to give the FDA and the USDA mandatory recall authority and the ability to fine violators. Urge Congress to establish "traceback" systems to enable the government and consumers to identify the source of the food responsible for a food-poisoning outbreak.

- Urge your congressional representatives to support funding for the FDA to increase inspection of food processors nationwide. The FDA inspects food plants every five years, and rarely checks imported food that enters the United States. The only solution is to fund more inspectors to check both domestic and imported foods for bacteria, parasites, pesticides, and other dangerous chemicals.

- Write and urge your congressional representatives to pass legislation requiring the USDA and the FDA to set limits on hazards in the food supply, such as bacteria, parasites, drug residues, and chemical hazards. Legislation should also require the food industry to conduct ongoing monitoring of its control systems, and fund government testing to audit the industry testing.

3. Reduce Animal Waste and Recycle It Safely

Twenty tons of animal waste is produced in the United States for every household in the country each year. If managed improperly, this waste could cause water pollution, noxious odors, and food poisoning.

Manure is the likely source of many of the hazards that cause food-poisoning outbreaks linked to fruits and vegetables. It frequently contains pathogens, such as *Salmonella, E. coli* O157:H7, *Campylobacter,* and *Listeria.* It also transmits parasites like *Cryptosporidium.* In addition, manure can contaminate wells that provide drinking water.

Despite those hazards, the treatment of manure is largely unregulated. Although organic producers now have standards for the use and application of manure in their operations, traditional farmers can use and dispose of manure in any manner that they find appropriate. Clearly, this needs to change. We need to urge the government and farmers to take action.

- Write to the EPA (401 M Street, S.W., Washington, D.C. 20460) and urge the agency to set standards for the application of manure on food crops. The EPA currently sets standards for the use of human sewage in agriculture, but has never adopted similar standards for animal manure. Composting manure or using digesters will reduce the pathogen levels. Applying manure six months or more before harvest would significantly reduce the risk.

- Encourage local farmers to use grazing techniques (like rotational grazing) that minimize the accumulation of large quantities of manure and to create centralized manure digesters in agricultural areas to compost manure and to capture the gases. These gases are an energy source that can be burned to produce heat and electricity.

- Require feedlots and other animal-containment facilities to operate manure-treatment facilities, comparable to those used for human sewage.

4. Fully Implement the Food Quality Protection Act

The Food Quality Protection Act holds great promise for reducing the levels of unsafe pesticides in our food. The 1996 law provides greater food-safety protections for children, requires the EPA to consider cumulative effects, and requires stores to give consumers more information on the pesticides in their products.

Now the challenge is to get the law implemented so that consumers can reap the benefits of safer food and safer pesticides. With over 20,000 pesticides approved for use today, the EPA has a big job to review these chemicals and ensure that they comply with the new law. Here are some steps you can take to encourage the EPA to keep pesticides high on its priority list.

- Write and call your representative and senators to tell them you support the Food Quality Protection Act. Make clear that you don't want the EPA to slow the implementation of an important law that will protect your children and future generations from harmful pesticides.

- Write to the EPA (401 M Street, S.W., Washington, D.C. 20460) and tell it to stop issuing emergency exemptions that allow pesticides to be used on food. These exemptions undermine the strong standards in the Food Quality Protection Act.

- Urge your congressional representatives to require the FDA and the USDA to conduct more tests for pesticide residues in domestic and imported foods. These tests should be combined with pathogen testing for fruits and vegetables. This increased testing would help keep contaminated foods off the market.

- Urge Congress to require the EPA to establish a centralized federal database that collects information on illnesses linked to pesticide exposure from states and make sure that your state is among those that require pesticide-illness reporting. Today only about 20 percent of the states require this reporting, including Arizona, California, Florida, Michigan, New Mexico, New York, Oregon, Texas, and Washington. Pesticide-illness reporting will help protect farmworkers and consumers from the improper use of pesticides.

- Urge farmers in your area to use alternatives to chemical pesticides, including crop rotation, natural predators, improved tilling, and other integrated pest-management techniques. These

techniques will help the environment while saving the farmers
money.

- Urge Congress to fund research and education efforts to help
  farmers develop and use safer alternatives to pesticides. More
  generally, the federally funded Sustainable Agriculture Research
  and Education Program (SARE) has been an effective, although
  embarrassingly underfunded, way to help farmers adopt
  environmentally friendly farming practices. Encourage Congress
  to significantly increase funding for the development of safe
  and environmentally beneficial genetically engineered fruits
  and vegetables that have been of little interest to
  companies.

5. Strengthen the Regulation of Genetically Modified Foods

For consumers, the key question about biotech foods is "Are they safe?"
Though the use of biotechnology in food production is still in its infancy,
the safety record so far provides some reassurance. To be honest, though, it
would be impossible to identify any long-term problems, such as immuno-
toxicity, cancer, or neurotoxicity.

Although existing genetically engineered foods may be safe, newer
products must be thoroughly tested and reviewed to ensure that they
don't cause allergic reactions or carry dangerous levels of naturally occurring toxins, such as solanine in potatoes. Although the FDA bears the
responsibility for ensuring the safety of genetically modified foods, the
FDA encourages, but does not require, companies to screen for such substances. In fact, companies are not even required to report the results of
their studies to the FDA.

In addition to food-safety concerns, genetically modified foods raise
ecological concerns. Many consumers worry about the effect of Bt corn
on butterflies and other nontarget organisms, the spread of genetically
engineered characteristics to wild relatives, or the development of pesticide resistance in insects or weeds. If used properly, genetically modified
foods could greatly benefit farmers, consumers, and the environment.
They hold out the promise of increased yields, reduced use of pesticides,
lower costs, and better nutrition. But, if misused, biotech foods could
cause great harm.

Here are steps you can take to improve government oversight of genetically engineered foods.

- Urge your senators and representative to strengthen the government's safety review of genetically engineered foods. All biotech food should go through a mandatory premarket *approval* process with specific data and testing requirements, along with an opportunity for public involvement. The National Academy of Sciences (NAS) should be commissioned to recommend precise assessment methods.

- Also tell Congress that it should close the current regulatory gaps to ensure that the products of biotechnology, from fast-growing fish to corn plants that produce industrial chemicals, receive thorough environmental reviews.

6. Create a Single Food-Safety Agency

Responsibility for overseeing the safety of our nation's food supply is divided among numerous federal agencies, including the USDA and the FDA, the Department of Commerce, and even the Treasury Department. The USDA is responsible for meat, including beef, poultry, and pork, while the FDA is responsible for every other type of food. But the Commerce Department operates a voluntary seafood-inspection program, and the Treasury Department oversees alcoholic beverages.

This system has created many inefficiencies and cracks through which food-safety problems can fall. For example, the USDA is responsible for the deadly *E. coli* bacteria on meat, while the FDA is responsible if it shows up on lettuce. Neither the USDA nor the FDA regulates food at the farm level (in fact, no agency does). The USDA and the EPA regulate the environmental impact of genetically modified foods, but the FDA oversees the safety aspects of most foods (except for what the EPA regulates). The EPA sets safety standards for pesticides in food, but the FDA enforces them. There are two systems for monitoring pesticide residues on fruits and vegetables, one at the FDA and the other at the USDA. Until recently, no agency was checking for pathogens on fruits and vegetables. And because of differences in goals, funding, and leadership among the USDA, the FDA, and the EPA, there are many other gaps in food-safety protections.

In addition, state and local governments have critical responsibilities to assure food safety locally, from inspecting local restaurants to food-poisoning-outbreak surveillance, but many of these state-run systems are voluntary and few are standardized.

The National Academy of Sciences has called for the consolidation of food-safety responsibility under a single statute, with a single budget and a single leader. The NAS's report, *Ensuring Safe Food from Production to Consumption,* concluded that the "current fragmented regulatory structure is not well equipped to meet the current challenges."[1]

The creation of a single food-safety agency that manages all food-safety issues at the federal level has been supported by many from the White House to Congress, from the General Accounting Office to Ralph Nader, from the Food Marketing Institute (FMI) to Consumers Union (the publisher of *Consumer Reports* magazine). Here's how you can help.

- Write or call your representative and senators and urge them to support efforts to create an independent food-safety agency. Tell them it is time to form a food-safety system in Washington that can truly protect consumers.

- Urge Congress to create a single system for inspecting all high-risk foods. Merge inspection functions and give the agency basic tools to enforce the laws. Create a single food-safety statute that would require the federal government to inspect foods based on the risk they pose to consumers.

CHAPTER NINE

PUTTING IT ALL TOGETHER: ADVICE FOR SAFE EATING

In this book, we've looked one at a time at the various health, safety, and environmental concerns associated with food. But when you are choosing what to eat, you don't have that luxury. You need to think about all of them together. How do you decide whether to eat cod, for example? Do you base your decision on the fact that it's good for your health, or that it's bad for the environment? Is it more important to worry about saturated fat, *Campylobacter,* pesticide residues, or global warming?

In this chapter, we summarize some of the key advice scattered throughout the book and show how it all fits together.

THE BIG PICTURE

The food Americans eat could be much safer, both for consumers and the environment. This book has discussed many problems, including an unbalanced, unhealthy diet; rising threats from deadly foodborne illnesses; widespread environmental degradation; and chemicals in foods. When all these problems are viewed together, a picture emerges of a food system requiring major reform.

As a consumer, you can protect yourself and move the food system in a positive direction through your food choices. In most cases, you don't have to choose between our advice on nutrition, food safety, and the environment. For example, cutting beef consumption both lowers the risk of heart disease and reduces water pollution.

In terms of personal health and safety, good nutrition should be the baseline standard for your food choices. The number of people who become seriously ill or die from eating a salt-, sugar-, fat-, and cholesterol-laden diet is many times greater than the number who die from a foodborne illness from bacteria, parasites, or viruses, or develop cancer from ingesting pesticides and other chemicals. While thousands die from food contaminated with pathogens, hundreds of thousands die from heart disease and stroke, which result in part from a poor diet. Others suffer from diabetes and other ailments. To maintain good health, sound nutrition should be the top food-related priority.

Foodborne illnesses and chemical intake are also important safety concerns, but they shouldn't cause you to stray from the principles of sound nutrition. Don't forgo vegetables and fruits because you are worried about *E. coli* or pesticides. Instead, you should consume as many vegetables and fruits as you can while taking steps, like washing produce thoroughly, that cut down on the risks.

Exposure to food contaminated with bacteria, viruses, and parasites poses a more immediate risk than food containing pesticides and other chemical residues. Eating a single food that contains deadly *E. coli, Salmonella,* or other pathogens can cause serious illness, sometimes leading to hospitalization or even death. Pesticides and other chemicals can lead to life-threatening cancer, but generally only after years of exposure, which means you don't need to be as vigilant every time you put something in your mouth. About 76 million Americans suffer from food poisoning each year, with an estimated 325,000 hospitalizations and 5,000 deaths. Pesticide poisoning is quite rare by comparison, although chronic exposure may cause as many as 6,000 cases of cancer each year.

Where does the environment fit into this hierarchy? Environmental action is in a different category because it focuses more on the societal benefits than personal ones. In most cases, however, consumers who make food choices that benefit the environment also help themselves. In fact, no single food-related action average Americans could take would have greater overall benefit, both for the environment and for their health, than to eat less meat. Next, purchasing organic foods not only helps the environment but lowers your chemical intake. The third main recommended environmental action—choosing sustainably caught fish—has no special health or food-safety advantages, but the inconvenience of avoiding certain types of seafood is small when compared with the considerable harm humans are causing fish species and ocean habitats.

Let's go through the various food categories to see how the different concerns play out.

Meat

We'll start with beef, chicken, and other meat. It is not big news that reducing meat consumption would significantly reduce consumption of saturated fat and cholesterol, thereby reducing the risk of heart disease and cancer of the colon and prostate. Meat is also frequently linked to foodborne illness, so reduced consumption would decrease the likelihood of such illness. Finally, it would benefit the environment more than any other single step.

Although most Americans should sharply reduce their meat intake, especially of beef and pork, many people will want to include some meat in their diets. Indeed, small amounts of meat will not cause major environmental or health problems, so long as it is prepared properly. Poultry is much better than red meat.

When you do eat meat, you can lower the health risks by cutting off the fat. This not only cuts your intake of artery-clogging saturated fat, but also of dioxins. You can lower the environmental impacts and help prevent the development of antibiotic-resistant bacteria by purchasing meat labeled organic or antibiotic-free.

You should also give careful attention to how you prepare meat, since almost all raw products carry one or more foodborne hazards. This means that raw meat and poultry should always be handled with the utmost caution, and we urge you to follow the recommendations for dealing with raw meat that we outlined in chapter 2. Be especially wary around ground beef and never eat an undercooked hamburger—or an undercooked piece of chicken, for that matter. Keep meat refrigerated, and don't eat any dishes containing meat that have been left out for more than two hours.

Dairy and Eggs

Fat content and *Salmonella* are the two most important concerns with dairy and eggs. To lower your intake of fat, restrict your consumption of egg yolks, butter, cream, cheese, and whole and 2 percent milk. To reduce the risk of food poisoning, handle unpasteurized eggs carefully:

don't eat them raw, keep them refrigerated, discard cracked ones, cook the yolks until firm, and use them within three weeks of purchase. Also avoid unpasteurized milk and raw-milk cheeses.

To lower environmental impacts, you can choose organic dairy products.

Fruits and Vegetables

For both your health and the environment, eat lots of fruits and vegetables. The National Cancer Institute recommends at least five servings a day, and you should consider that a minimum.

But after that, things get more complicated. Processed fruits and vegetables are much less likely to harbor harmful bacteria and viruses than fresh ones, but they often suffer from reduced taste and nutritional quality. Although organic fruits and vegetables are better than conventionally grown produce for the environment and carry fewer chemical residues, they still may be contaminated with pathogens. So here's what we recommend.

- Do NOT restrict your intake of fruits and vegetables because of concern about disease or chemical residues. Do NOT avoid fresh produce.

- Eat more of those vegetables that are nutritionally superior, like spinach, sweet potato, and red pepper.

- Always rinse fresh fruits and vegetables under running water. Whenever possible, first wash the produce in a bowl of water that includes a few drops of dish soap before rinsing it under cold running water. You can also peel fruits and vegetables.

- Buy organic produce, but take the same precautions as you would with conventional produce. Give special preference to organic fruits and vegetables when the price differential is small or when the conventional alternatives are high in pesticide residues (e.g., peaches and frozen winter squash).

- Make a special effort to buy organic fruits that your young children consume in large quantities (e.g., apple juice, apples, pears).

- If you can, grow some of your own fruits or vegetables organically, or purchase some from local farms you trust.

- Avoid alfalfa sprouts, unpasteurized apple cider, and other minimally processed foods that have a poor safety record.

Grains

For your health, select whole grains over refined ones, like white flour. Choose whole-wheat bread, brown rice, and whole grain cereals, such as oatmeal, raisin bran, and shredded wheat.

For the environment, choose organic grains.

Seafood

There is a lot to think about when choosing fish and other seafood. From a nutrition standpoint, they are generally good choices, as long as you avoid unhealthy preparation techniques such as deep-frying. But you need to worry about everything else. Some, like Gulf Coast oysters and barracuda, can cause serious illness. Others, like shark and Great Lakes region carp, contain levels of mercury or PCBs that may be especially harmful to pregnant women and small children. Eating others, like Chilean sea bass and orange roughy, causes unacceptably high environmental harm.

Labeling may eventually help you sort through the myriad seafood choices, but in the meantime, there is no alternative to trying to keep track of which ones pose risks and which are safe. Figure 101 summarizes some of the seafood choices to avoid, although we suggest you go back to read chapters 2, 3, and 4 for more information on them.

Snacks

Because they are so highly processed, you won't find harmful pathogens in packaged snacks. But you will find lots of empty calories with little nutritional value, so stay away from snacks loaded with salt, sugar, and saturated fat. By making it a habit to always read the nutrition label before purchasing a packaged snack, you will be reminded of the large quantities of calories, fat, and salt in just one serving and may have an easier time resisting temptation. (The same label-reading habit makes sense for processed foods other than snacks.) Also, don't get suckered into buying a snack just because it says "organic" on the label, since that doesn't necessarily mean that it has any fewer empty calories.

To make it easier to resist unhealthy snacks, keep a handy supply of easy-to-eat healthy ones, such as baby carrots and easy-to-pack fruits.

Drinks

Most likely you consume more tap water than any other liquid. Therefore, as we described in chapter 4, find out whether your water is safe
to drink. But don't assume that bottled water is safer, because it may
not be.

In terms of nutrition, avoid soft drinks with lots of empty calories.
They are a main cause of weight gain. Instead, choose water, low-fat
milk, seltzer, or fruit juice.

Alcoholic beverages appear to help protect against heart disease if
consumed in moderate quantities (one drink a day for women; two for

FIGURE 10
SEAFOOD TO AVOID

High environmental damage	Risk of foodborne illness	High mercury, dioxin, or PCB levels—avoid large quantities, small quantities OK (especially a concern for pregnant women and children)
Atlantic swordfish	Raw shellfish, especially from Gulf Coast waters	Shark
Chilean sea bass (Patagonian toothfish)	Barracuda	Swordfish
Cod	Grouper, amberjack, and red snapper from southern Florida, Hawaii, and tropical waters	King mackerel
Orange roughy	Smoked fish (for pregnant women and the elderly)	Tuna
Pacific rockfish (rock cod)		White and golden snapper
Red snapper		Fish caught in rivers, lakes, and streams, especially in the Great Lakes region
Shark		

men). But don't start drinking alcohol for this reason. Also, many people should not drink even moderate amounts, including those with a family history of alcohol abuse, pregnant women, and young people. And if you drink coffee, choosing types labeled organic, Bird Friendly, Eco-OK, or Fair Trade has environmental benefits.

Eating Out

It's always tempting to abandon good nutritional sense when you eat out, so you should choose carefully. Look for restaurants and takeouts where you can include vegetables and fruits in your meal. Stay away from fried foods and other items loaded with calories, saturated fat, *trans* fat, and salt. And perhaps more than anything, don't eat more than you need or want to just because restaurant portions are overly large. Instead, decide how much is appropriate and bring the rest home.

To cut down on the risk of foodborne illness, avoid poorly monitored warming trays in take-out bars and other food services that leave meats, egg products, and other heated foods out for many hours between 40 and 140 degrees.

CONCLUSION

We've given you a lot to remember, but by taking a little care in what you buy and heeding a few sensible precautions, you can protect yourself and improve the environment. By feeling good about your choices, eating will be a pleasurable experience.

Of course, it would be nice if all food was perfectly safe. A little time spent trying to influence government policy can help bring us closer to this goal. And remember that every time you buy food, you are voting with your dollars. Try to make choices that will point the food industry toward a safer system.

Finally, we don't want to pretend that this book is the final word on the safety of your food. While many of our recommendations should remain valid for years to come, the food system is changing fast—in some ways that are reducing risks and in others that are adding new ones. So it's important to keep up on the latest developments. The websites and periodicals listed in this book's resource guide (Appendix B) should help you do that.

Safe eating!

APPENDIX A

A WEEK'S FOOD

When all the food that is sold to food stores, restaurants, and other food service establishments is tallied up and divided by the number of people in the country, we end up with the results below for a week's food production for an average American. Of course, some people use more of particular items, while others use less. For example, small children usually eat less than adults and rarely consume coffee or beer. Not all of the food listed below is eaten, since some of it is wasted, either in the home, en route, or in the store or restaurant. You might compare your own food consumption for a week to this profile of an average American.

The data below is derived from information in the U.S. Census Bureau's *Statistical Abstract of the United States: 2000* (Washington, D.C.: U.S. Government Printing Office, 2000), pp. 147–148, which in turn bases its tables on data from the U.S. Department of Agriculture.

Red meat (boneless, trimmed weight)	**2 lbs. 4 oz.**
Beef	1 lb. 4 oz.
Pork	15 oz.
Lamb and veal	0.5 oz.
Poultry (boneless, trimmed weight)	**1 lb. 4 oz.**
Chicken	1 lb.
Turkey	4 oz.
Fish and shellfish (boneless, trimmed weight)	**5 oz.**
Eggs	**4.7 eggs**
Dairy products (milk equivalent weight)	**11 lbs. 3 oz.**
Milk and flavored milks	1.8 quarts
Cheese	9 oz.
Ice cream and other frozen dairy desserts	9 oz.
Cream, sour cream, cream dips	3 oz.
Condensed and evaporated milk	2 oz.

Yogurt	1 oz.
Cottage cheese	1 oz.

Fats and oils   **1 lb. 4 oz.**

Flour, rice, corn, and other cereal products   **3 lbs. 12 oz.**
Wheat flour	2 lbs. 13 oz.
Corn products	7 oz.
Rice	6 oz.
Oats and other	2 oz.

Sweeteners   **3 lbs.**
Corn sweeteners	1 lb. 11 oz.
Sugar (cane, beet)	1 lb. 5 oz.
Honey, maple syrup, and others	0.4 oz.

Fruits (farm weight)   **5 lbs. 7 oz.**
Fruit juices	1.1 quarts
Fresh fruits	2 lbs. 8 oz.
Frozen, dried, and canned fruits	11 oz.

Vegetables, beans, and potatoes (farm weight)   **8 lbs. 2 oz.**
Frozen, canned, and other processed	4 lbs. 3 oz.
Fresh vegetables	2 lbs. 11 oz.
Potatoes	15 oz.
Potatoes for chips	5 oz.

Selected beverages*
Carbonated soft drinks	4.1 quarts
Beer	2.6 quarts
Milk and flavored milks	1.8 quarts
Coffee	1.8 quarts
Bottled water	1.0 quart
Tea	0.6 quart
Fruit drinks	0.6 quart
Wine	0.2 quart
Distilled spirits	0.2 quart
Bottled iced tea	0.1 quart

---

* The sugar and corn sweeteners in these drinks are also included in the sweetener category above. Milk and flavored milks are also included in the dairy products category above.

Other

Cocoa beans	2 oz.
Peanuts	2 oz.
Tree nuts (shelled)	0.7 oz.

APPENDIX B

RESOURCES FOR EATING SAFELY

BOOKS

Many books and reports have been written on topics related to food safety, nutrition, and the environmental impacts of food production. Here we focus on ones that can provide you with practical information, as well as a few others that we find especially interesting.

Brower, Michael, and Warren Leon. *The Consumer's Guide to Effective Environmental Choices: Practical Advice from the Union of Concerned Scientists*. New York: Three Rivers Press, 1999. A clear, practical, and scientifically sound overview of the relationship between consumers and the environment. Some of the environmental data in *Is Our Food Safe?* was derived from the analysis for this book.

Charles, Daniel. *Lords of the Harvest: Biotech, Big Money, and the Future of Food*. Cambridge, Mass.: Perseus Publishing, 2001. The behind-the-scenes story of the development of genetically engineered crops.

Cutler, Karan Davis, et al. *Burpee: The Complete Vegetable and Herb Gardener: A Guide to Growing Your Garden Organically*. New York: Macmillan, 1997. This comprehensive, beautifully illustrated volume is one of the best of the many good books on growing vegetables organically.

Jacobson, Michael F., and Bruce Maxwell. *What Are We Feeding Our Kids?* New York: Workman Publishing, 1994. An excellent source for information on children's nutrition.

Kiple, Kenneth, and Kriemhild Conee Ornelas. *The Cambridge World History of Food*. 2 vols. New York: Cambridge University Press, 2000. This mammoth compendium of articles from more than 200 leading food experts from around the world covers thousands of years of people's changing eating, cooking, and farming practices. It includes a dictionary of all the plants people eat.

Kramer, Mark. *Three Farms: Making Milk, Meat, and Money from the American Soil.* Boston: Little Brown, 1980. Although a bit outdated, this beautifully crafted book's evocative portraits of a Massachusetts dairy farm, an Iowa corn-hog farm, and a California agribusiness reveal the challenges faced by family farmers and the problems with corporate agriculture.

Layne, Scott, et al. *Firepower in the Lab: Automation in the Fight Against Infectious Diseases and Bioterrorism.* Washington, D.C.: Joseph Henry Press, 2001. A timely report on action that can be taken to protect against bioterrorism.

Lee, Mercedes, et al. *Seafood Lover's Almanac.* Islip, N.Y.: National Audubon Society's Living Oceans Program, 2000. A well-illustrated, fish-by-fish guide to a wide range of seafood, providing information on each type's appearance, habits, nutritional content, and environmental status. The book recommends which to buy and which to avoid, and includes interesting recipes.

Masumoto, David Mas. *Epitaph for a Peach: Four Seasons on My Family Farm.* San Francisco: HarperSanFrancisco, 1995. A movingly written memoir of the challenges faced by an environmentally oriented family farmer trying to grow unusual fruit when the food system emphasizes standardization.

McHughen, Alan. *Pandora's Picnic Basket: The Potential and Hazards of Genetically Modified Foods.* New York: Oxford University Press, 2000. A solid, understandable overview of the science of genetically engineered foods. It underplays some of their environmental risks.

Nestle, Marion. *Food Politics: How the Food Industry Influences Nutrition and Health.* Berkeley: University of California Press, 2002. A disturbing exposé of the food industry's marketing and lobbying efforts to influence government policy.

Robbins, John. *The Food Revolution: How Your Diet Can Save Your Life and Your World.* Berkeley, Calif.: Conari Press, 2001. The latest from the author of *Diet for a New America.* Robbins catalogs problems associated with meat production and makes the case for vegetarian eating. His critique of biotechnology is overblown.

Safina, Carl. *Song for the Blue Ocean: Encounters Along the World's Coasts and Beneath the Seas.* New York: Henry Holt, 1998. Safina takes readers on an engrossing tour of the world's oceans to show the damage humans are causing by fishing and other activities.

Satin, Mortin. *Food Alert! The Ultimate Sourcebook for Food Safety.* New York: Checkmark Books, 1999. A comprehensive discussion of foodborne diseases, with advice to consumers on safe handling of food.

Schlosser, Eric. *Fast Food Nation: The Dark Side of the All-American Meal.* Boston: Houghton Mifflin, 2001. While exposing the pernicious influence of the fast-food industry on the American economy and society, the author entertainingly discusses the history and current state of fast-food franchises, cattle ranching, teenage workers, multinational food corporations, food additives, conditions in meatpacking plants, and Americans' diets.

Steingraber, Sandra. *Living Downstream: A Scientist's Personal Investigation of Cancer and the Environment.* Rev. ed. New York: Vintage Books, 1998. The author, a biologist and a cancer survivor, links high cancer rates in the farming region of rural Illinois and elsewhere to the use of pesticides and other chemicals. An engrossing story with accessible scientific information.

Teitel, Martin, and Kimberly A. Wilson. *Genetically Engineered Food: Changing the Nature of Nature.* Rev. ed. Rochester, Vt.: Park Street Press, 2001. This book clearly and concisely presents the critics' case against biotechnology.

United Nations Development Programme (UNDP) et al. *World Resources, 2000–2001: People and Ecosystems, the Fraying Web of Life.* Washington, D.C.: World Resources Institute, 2000. Several authoritative international agencies assess the condition of the global environment, including agricultural ecosystems, ocean fisheries, and coastal areas affected by farming and fishing. Includes statistical tables with data on all the world's nations.

PERIODICALS

Nutrition Action Healthletter. Lively monthly newsletter dispenses advice from the Center for Science in the Public Interest. Each issue includes ratings of consumer products, along with examples of "food porn" and the "right stuff."

Organic Gardening. Published by Rodale, this is the world's best-selling gardening magazine. It has been showing readers how to garden chemical-free since 1942.

Outbreak Alert. A periodic report by the Center for Science in the Public Interest on foodborne-poisoning outbreaks in the United States during the last decade.

WEBSITES

Literally thousands of websites cover one or more of the topics discussed in this book. Here are a few of the sites that we believe are especially interesting and useful to the general public.

General

Center for Science in the Public Interest
www.cspinet.org
CSPI's website covers nutrition, food safety, genetically engineered foods, antibiotic resistance, and food additives. It includes consumer advice, nutrition quizzes, short fact sheets, full reports, legislative updates, background information, the latest food news, and selected articles from *Nutrition Action Healthletter.*

Consumers Union
www.consumersunion.org
A consumer advocacy website from the publisher of *Consumer Reports.* It includes background information, reports, and legislative updates on a wide range of food-safety-related topics, including food contaminants, pesticides, mad cow disease, organic foods, and genetically engineered foods.

Consumers Union Guide to Environmental Labels
www.eco-labels.org
A handy description, analysis, and evaluation of dozens of different certification labels placed on foods by governments and private certify-

ing organizations. It also evaluates such general claims as "free range," "natural," and "no artificial ingredients."

Food and Drug Administration
www.fda.gov
The FDA describes its programs to regulate foods and provides background information on foodborne illness, dietary supplements, nutrition, and other topics.

Nutrition.gov and FoodSafety.gov
www.nutrition.gov and www.foodsafety.gov
Two entryways to numerous government websites on food, nutrition, and food safety. They cover everything from nutrition labels and general food facts to home canning and dietary supplements. If you don't know which government agency to turn to for information, these websites are the best starting points.

U.S. Department of Agriculture
www.usda.gov
This government department provides up-to-date news releases, information on hot topics, and a description of its programs. Among the useful site features are food-safety tips from the Partnership for Food Safety Education, information about the agency's new organic-food labels, and the government perspective on genetically engineered foods.

Environmental Impacts

EarthSave
www.earthsave.org
This membership organization's website provides information on the environmental, nutritional, and animal-rights reasons for reducing meat consumption. It includes links to many other healthy-eating and vegetarian websites, some with recipes.

Environmental Defense
www.environmentaldefense.org
This environmental advocacy organization offers fact sheets, reports, and news releases on the status of various marine and land-based ecosystems. It covers such topics as antibiotic resistance, aquaculture, and genetically engineered foods. It has a brief list of seafood to avoid and seafood to choose.

Natural Resources Defense Council
www.nrdc.org
Another environmental advocacy organization that provides fact sheets, reports, and news releases. This website has solid, readable material on water use and water pollution from agriculture, drinking water, factory farms, pesticides, and sustainable agriculture. It also has a brief list of seafood yeas and nays.

Union of Concerned Scientists
www.ucsusa.org
This national advocacy organization's user-friendly website offers non-technical background information on sustainable agriculture, antibiotic use in livestock, and the environmental risks of genetically engineered foods, as well as news about current government policies.

U.S. Environmental Protection Agency
www.epa.gov
Information on the environmental impacts of food production are scattered throughout the EPA's website. Especially interesting and useful features include local drinking water information (www.epa.gov/safewater/dwinfo.htm) and interactive practical advice for consumers on pesticides and food (www.gov/pesticides/food).

Food Safety

Centers for Disease Control and Prevention
www.cdc.gov
This government agency provides disease-by-disease fact sheets on food-borne illnesses organized around frequently asked questions. It also offers advice on how to avoid those illnesses and statistics on their prevalence.

FoodHACCP
www.foodhaccp.com
This site provides links to news and information on food-safety topics, including pathogens and BSE. Free subscription required.

Keep Antibiotics Working
www.keepantibioticsworking.com
The best site for the use of antibiotics in agriculture. Sponsored by leading health and environmental advocacy groups, it encourages visitors to send e-mails to government and industry officials.

Penn State Food Safety
http://foodsafety.cas.psu.edu
The Pennsylvania State University Department of Food Science has created a website with news updates and consumer advice on safe methods for cooking, storing, and preserving food. Includes over 1,300 links to online food-safety resources.

Genetically Engineered Foods

Ag Biotech InfoNet
www.biotech-info.net
This site collects research summaries and opinion articles from magazines and newspapers around the world.

Food Biotechnology Communications Network
www.foodbiotech.org
Canadian government agencies and biotech companies support this consumer-oriented compendium of the latest biotechnology news. It includes a user-friendly database of frequently asked questions.

Information Systems for Biotech
www.isb.vt.edu
Similar to the Ag Biotech InfoNet website, but it tends to be more favorable toward biotechnology.

National Academy of Sciences
www.nas.edu
The National Academy's Board on Agriculture and Natural Resources produces sophisticated, well-balanced, but technical reports on the complex environmental and public health issues raised by genetically engineered foods.

See also the websites of the Center for Science in the Public Interest, Consumers Union, Food First, International Food Policy Research Institute, and Union of Concerned Scientists listed elsewhere in this appendix.

International Food Supply

Food and Agriculture Organization

www.fao.org

This UN agency reports on global trends, promotes sustainable agriculture, and disseminates information from its many conferences and reports. This is the best starting point for finding out what's going on around the world in farming, fishing, and aquaculture.

Food First

www.foodfirst.org

The Institute for Food and Development Policy, better known as Food First, promotes reform of the global food system. It makes the case that biotechnology could be harmful to poor farmers in developing countries.

Future Harvest

www.futureharvest.org

A public education effort organized by 16 food-research centers around the world, it provides information about the importance of food production and the ways in which improved agriculture could reduce hunger and environmental damage. One of the centers, the International Food Policy Research Institute, has its own website (www.ifpri.org), which assesses the prospects for the global food supply and analyzes policies for meeting the world's food needs.

Nutrition

American Dietetic Association

www.eatright.org

This site provides user-friendly information on healthy lifestyle, diet, and nutrition choices. It features daily health tips and a "Find a Dietician" link.

Cyberdiet

www.cyberdiet.com

A lively site with interactive assessment tools for planning a healthy diet and evaluating different meals.

Tufts Nutrition Navigator

www.navigator.tufts.edu

Descriptions and ratings of hundreds of websites by Tufts University nutritionists.

Organic Foods

Community Supported Agriculture
www.csacenter.org
Information about the Community Supported Agriculture (CSA) movement and a directory of CSA farms across the country.

National Organic Program
www.ams.usda.gov/nop/
This site provides background information on the government's organic program and links to other sites related to organic agriculture.

Organic Consumers Association
www.purefood.org
An extensive database of articles, news reports, and links for activists and consumers. It focuses on the benefits of organic food and the dangers of biotechnology and industrial agriculture. The website also provides an opportunity for consumers to get involved in various campaigns.

Organic Trade Association
www.ota.com
The business association of the organic industry has a website with a searchable directory of its member farms and companies, as well as background information on organic foods.

International Federation of Organic Agriculture Movements
www.ifoam.org
The website of the umbrella organization for national and local organic groups reports on the latest trends, developments, and research worldwide.

Pesticides

Consumers Union Paradox Theatre
www.ecologic-ipm.com
Part of a project to ensure that the Food Quality Protection Act is implemented on schedule and reduces human exposure to pesticides.

Environmental Working Group's Food News
www.FoodNews.org
User-friendly news and information about pesticides in foods from a national advocacy organization. An interactive virtual supermarket allows users to find out which pesticides are found on a wide range of specific foods.

Pesticide Action Network
www.panna.org
News, reports, and background information from an antipesticide advocacy coalition. It includes a database that describes each pesticide's toxicity and regulatory status.

Seafood

American Oceans Campaign
www.americanoceans.org
Summaries of the latest fish research in nontechnical language, information about efforts to protect ocean habitats, and suggestions on what you can do to help.

Marine Stewardship Council
www.msc.org
This independent international organization, which certifies sustainable fisheries, explains its certification process, and provides information for consumers about buying seafood and the state of the world's fisheries.

Monterey Bay Aquarium
www.mbayaq.org
This California aquarium presents interesting background information about the world's endangered oceans and sustainable fishing. It offers a user-friendly seafood guide with clear explanations about why certain types of seafood are recommended or disapproved.

National Audubon Society
www.audubon.org/campaign/lo
The website of Audubon's Living Oceans Program features the organization's downloadable Seafood Guide; news related to fisheries and other marine issues; and ways in which citizens can help protect threatened marine life.

Seafood Choices Alliance
www.seafoodchoices.com
Although this new organization seeks to provide fishermen, chefs, and seafood merchants with information about sound seafood choices, its website is also of interest to consumers. Its database includes the environmental ratings other groups have given to various kinds of seafood.

APPENDIX C

ABOUT THE CENTER FOR SCIENCE IN THE PUBLIC INTEREST

For 30 years, the Center for Science in the Public Interest (CSPI) has been a strong advocate for good nutrition, food safety, improved alcohol policies, and sound science. CSPI helped put the Nutrition Facts label on all food products, supported changes to meat and poultry inspection that significantly reduced *Salmonella* contamination, lobbied for the new U.S. Department of Agriculture (USDA) organic label, obtained restrictions on unsafe additives, fought for warning labels on alcoholic beverages, and improved food labeling, including getting the government to require safe-handling notices on packages of meat, poultry, and eggs.

In 1971, three young scientists founded CSPI, a unique organization formed to provide expertise on behalf of consumers on a broad range of environmental and health issues. In the mid-1970s, CSPI zeroed in on nutrition and food safety. The significant impact of poor nutrition on health made it urgent that an aggressive public-interest organization take up this challenge.

The urgency derived from the gravity of the diseases that the American diet was causing: heart disease, cancers, stroke, diabetes, hypertension, and obesity. Unhealthy eating, together with lack of physical activity, causes about half a million premature deaths each year. Better nutrition could save more than $71 billion annually.

CSPI also works to reduce the toll of foodborne illnesses. One of CSPI's highest priorities is strong federal food-safety, food-inspection, and food-additive laws. The nation's long-established food-safety systems were not designed to address today's challenges, like bacteria, mad cow disease, and genetically modified foods. Meat, poultry, and seafood inspection in the United States is archaic. As a result, inspectors have little chance of detecting dangerous bacteria that contaminate the food supply.

In the late 1990s, CSPI worked with the USDA to improve the inspection system for meat and poultry and persuaded Congress to add more than $220 million to the federal food-safety budget. That new funding has meant more inspectors, more inspections, and safer food. As a result, rates of *Salmonella* contamination in meat and poultry have declined dramatically.

But large gaps still exist in the food-safety net, and they must be closed. Most foods are not tested for hazards prior to being sold to the public. So CSPI has petitioned the government to test more foods for more hazards, like checking ready-to-eat meats for *Listeria,* poultry for *Campylobacter,* and beef carcasses for *E. coli* O157:H7.

CSPI continually watches for emerging hazards in the food supply and urges the government to take action to protect the public. For example, ensuring that mad cow disease (bovine spongiform encephalopathy) does not appear on our shores is a top priority. The USDA and the FDA have been unusually vigilant in their job of guarding America's cattle population from this disease. And CSPI has been a driving force behind some of the critical safeguards against the human form of the disease. We helped to stop the stunning of cattle by air-injection rifles, which was contaminating meat with potentially infective brain tissue. We also urged the USDA to establish procedures for keeping spinal cords out of meat.

For the latest on nutrition and food safety, you can join CSPI for $24 annually and receive the *Nutrition Action Healthletter,* the largest-circulation newsletter in the country. It is an award-winning, 16-page illustrated newsletter that is published 10 times a year. It provides reliable information on nutrition and food safety, debunks deceptive ads, and gives you the lowdown on contaminants in your food.

Beyond giving you information to help you improve your health, CSPI serves as your lobbyist and watchdog in Washington, where we will continue to work to achieve political reforms. We hope you'll join the 800,000 other concerned citizens who are CSPI members.

Center for Science in the Public Interest
1875 Connecticut Ave., N.W., Suite 300
Washington, D.C. 20009
(202) 332-9110
www.cspinet.org

NOTES

Chapter One. If Our Food Is So Safe, Why Are We Worried?

1. Daniel J. Boorstin, *The Americans: The Democratic Experience* (New York: Random House, 1973), p. 314.
2. Stephen Nissenbaum, *Sex, Diet, and Debility in Jacksonian America: Sylvester Graham and Health Reform* (Westport, Conn.: Greenwood Press, 1980), p. 6.
3. World Health Organization, *World Health Report 2001* (Geneva, Switz.: World Health Organization, 2001), p. 144.
4. For an interesting discussion of Americans' attitudes toward food-safety risks, see a paper by Edward Groth III, *Risk Communication in the Context of Consumer Perceptions of Risk* (Yonkers, N.Y.: Consumers Union, 1998).
5. For background on topsoil and erosion, see James E. Horne and Maura McDermott, *The Next Green Revolution: Essential Steps to a Healthy, Sustainable Agriculture* (New York: Food Products Press, 2001), pp. 67–93.
6. National Agricultural Statistics Service, *USDA Historical Track Records* (Washington, D.C.: U.S. Department of Agriculture, 2001), available at www.usda.gov/nass/pubs/histdata.htm.
7. Marion Nestle and Michael Jacobson, "Halting the Obesity Epidemic: A Public Health Policy Approach," *Public Health Report* (January/February 2000), p. 16.
8. Personal communication from Margo Wootan, Center for Science in the Public Interest, January 14, 2002.
9. Bonnie Liebman and David Schardt, "Diet and Health: Ten Megatrends," *Nutrition Action Healthletter* (January/February 2001), p. 12.
10. Quoted in Nestle and Jacobson, "Obesity Epidemic," p. 19.
11. Ibid.
12. Department of Agriculture, "Briefing Room: Diet and Health: Food Consumption and Nutrient Intake Tables," Food Consumption Table 5, available at www.ers.usda.gov/briefing/DietAndHealth/data.

Chapter Two. Bugs, More Bugs, and Superbugs:
Handling Hazards in Our Food

1. Statement of David Satcher, Director of Centers for Disease Control and Prevention, before the Committee on Government Reform and Oversight, Subcommittee on Human Resources and Intergovernmental Relations, U.S. House of Representatives, May 23, 1996, pp. 11–12.

2. Testimony of Roni Rudolph, S.T.O.P.!—Safe Tables Our Priority, Symposium for Congress and the Media on Foodborne Illness, Washington, D.C., September 21, 1993.

3. Morton Satin, *Food Alert! The Ultimate Sourcebook for Food Safety* (New York: Checkmark Books, 1999), pp. 184–187.

4. Rudolph testimony.

5. Statement of State of Washington Department of Health, "State Health Officials Confirm *E. coli* Bacterium in Ground Beef," Olympia, Washington, January 17, 1993.

6. Personal communication (e-mail) from Bert Bartleson, January 22, 2001.

7. Rudolph testimony.

8. "Foodborne Illness: What Consumers Need to Know," fact sheet, USDA and FDA, distributed August 2000 for use in September 2000 as part of the International Food Safety Council's National Food Safety Education Month.

9. Paul S. Mead et al., "Food-Related Illness and Death in the United States," *Emerging Infectious Diseases* 5, no. 5 (1999).

10. Satin, *Food Alert!,* pp. 110–111.

11. Caroline Smith DeWaal et al., *Outbreak Alert! Closing the Gaps in Our Federal Food-Safety Net* (Washington D.C.: Center for Science in the Public Interest, updated and revised October 2001), pp. 1, 16–43.

12. Telephone conversation with Laurie Girand, mother of Anna Girand, December 7, 2000.

13. Centers for Disease Control and Prevention, "Ten Public Health Achievements—Safer and Healthier Foods," available at www.phppo.cdc.gov/phtn/tenachievements/food1/food1.asp.

14. Upton Sinclair, *The Jungle* (New York: Bantam Books, 1906).

15. Guy Gugliotta, "Meat Inspection Agency Faces Reorganization—New Food Safety Standards Prompt Structural Overhaul," *Washington Post,* July 26, 1996, p. A25.

16. Food Safety and Inspection Service, *Progress Report on Salmonella Testing of Raw Meat and Poultry Products* (Washington, D.C.: Food Safety and In-

spection Service, March 2000), available at www.fsis.usda.gov/OA/background/salmtest5.htm.

17. Centers for Disease Control and Prevention, "Update: Multistate Outbreak of Listeriosis—United States, 1998–1999," *Morbidity and Mortality Weekly Report* 47, no. 51 (January 8, 1999), pp. 1117–1118.

18. Caroline Smith DeWaal et al., *Unexpected Consequences: Miscarriage and Birth Defects from Tainted Food* (Washington, D.C.: Center for Science in the Public Interest, January 2000), p. 3.

19. Mead et al., "Food-Related Illness and Death," p. 611, Table 3; Council for Agricultural Science and Technology, *Foodborne Pathogens: Risks and Consequences,* Task Force Report no. 122 (1994), p. 45; Jordan Tappero et al., "Reduction in the Incidence of Human Listeriosis in the United States: Effectiveness of Prevention Efforts?" *Journal of the American Medical Association* 273, no. 14 (1995), p. 1118.

20. Smith DeWaal et al., *Unexpected Consequences,* p. 9.

21. "Turkey Basics: Handling Precooked Dinners," Food Safety and Inspection Service, United States Department of Agriculture, Food Safety Facts, Information for Consumers, rev. November 2000, available at www.fsis.usda.gov/oa/pubs/tbtakeout.htm.

22. Mississippi State University Extension Service, "Feeding a Crowd? Do It Safely," last modified October 2, 2001, available at http://msucares.com/pubs/is645.htm.

23. "USDA Urges Consumers to Use Food Thermometer When Cooking Ground Beef Patties," News Release, Department of Agriculture, Food Safety and Inspection Service, August 11, 1998.

24. Department of Agriculture, Food Safety and Inspection Service, The Thermy™ Campaign, Food Thermometers and Food Temperature Indicators, updated November 29, 2001, available at www.fsis.usda.gov/oa/thermy/ktherms.htm.

25. "USDA Offers Advice for Preparing a Safe Thanksgiving Meal," Department of Agriculture, Food Safety and Inspection Service, USDA News Release no. 0457.99; National Turkey Federation, "Turkey Basics: Handling Cooked Dinners," available at http://www.eatturkey.com/consumer/cookinfo/dinners.html; "Staphylococcal Food Poisoning from Turkey at a Country Club Buffet—New Mexico," *MMWR Weekly* 35, no. 46 (November 21, 1986), 715–716, 721–722.

26. "USDA Offers Advice for Preparing a Safe Thanksgiving Meal."

27. Ibid.

28. Satin, *Food Alert!,* p. 242.

29. Stephen F. Dealler et al., "Transmissible Spongiform Encephalopathies:

The Threat of BSE to Man," *Food Microbiology* 7 (1990), pp. 253–279; Conversation between Oprah Winfrey and Howard Lyman of the Humane Society of the United States, April 16, 1996, *The Oprah Show*.

30. John Darnton, "Britain Ties Deadly Brain Disease to Cow Ailment," *New York Times,* March 21, 1996, p. A1.

31. World Health Organization Information Fact Sheet no. 113, rev. June 2001, available at www.who.int.inf-fs/en/fact113.html; "USDA Actions to Prevent Bovine Spongiform Encephalopathy (BSE)," FAS Online, available at www.fas.usda.gov/dlp/BSE/aphischron.html.

32. "McDonald's First-Quarter Net Fell 16% Due to Concerns About Mad-Cow Disease," *Wall Street Journal,* April 20, 2001, p. B8; British Ministry of Agriculture, Fisheries and Food, The Specified Bovine Offal (Amendment) Order, 1995 no. 3246; European Commission, Health and Consumer Protection Directorate, "Commission Approves Further Protection Measures Against BSE," general press release, Brussels, February 7, 2001, available at www.europa.eu.int/comm/dgs/health_consumer/library/press/press106_en.html.

33. Patricia B. Lieberman and Margo G. Wootan, *Protecting the Crown Jewels of Medicine—a Strategic Plan to Preserve the Effectiveness of Antibiotics* (Washington, D.C.: Center for Science in the Public Interest, 1998), p. 1.

34. Margaret Mellon et al., *Hogging It: Estimates of Antimicrobial Abuse in Livestock* (Cambridge, Mass.: Union of Concerned Scientists, January 2001), p. xiii. Even if this estimate turns out to be high, it cannot be questioned that animal use of antibiotics dwarfs human use.

35. Lieberman and Wootan, *Protecting the Crown Jewels,* p. 12.

36. Letter to David A. Kessler, Commissioner of FDA, from David Satcher, Director of CDC, August 16, 1995.

37. Food and Drug Administration (FDA), "Enrofloxacin for Poultry: Opportunity for Hearing," Notice, *Federal Register* 65, no. 211 (October 31, 2000), pp. 64954–64955.

38. S. Rossiter et al., "High Prevalence of Antimicrobial-Resistant, Including Fluoroquinolone-Resistant, *Campylobacter* on Chicken in U.S. Grocery Stores," 100th General Meeting of the American Society for Microbiology, poster C296, Los Angeles, May 24, 2000; FDA, "Enrofloxacin," p. 64955.

39. Frank Møller Aarestrup et al. "Effect of Abolishment of the Use of Antimicrobial Agents for Growth Promotion on Occurrence of Antimicrobial Resistance in Fecal Enterococci from Food Animals in Denmark," *Antimicrobial Agents and Chemotherapy* 45, no. 7 (July 2001), pp. 2054–2059. On the U.S. government's approach, see Interagency Task Force on Antimicrobial Resistance, *A Public Health Action Plan to Combat Antimicrobial Resistance, Part 1: Domestic Issues* (Washington, D.C.: Interagency Task

Force on Antimicrobial Resistance, 2001), available at www.cdc.gov/drugresistance/actionplan/aractionplan.pdf.

40. Pat Leidl et al., *Overcoming Antimicrobial Resistance* (Geneva, Switz.: World Health Organization, 2000), Chap. 5, available at www.who.int/infectious-disease-report/2000/ch5.htm.

41. Pam Belluck and Christopher Drew, "Tracing Bout of Illness to Small Lettuce Farm," *New York Times,* January 5, 1998.

42. Smith DeWaal et al. *Outbreak Alert!,* pp. 1, 16, 31–34.

43. Guodong Wang et al., "Fate of Enterohemorrhagic *Escherichia coli* 0157:H7 in Bovine Feces," *Applied and Environmental Microbiology* (July 1996), pp. 2567–2570.

44. "FDA Advises Consumers about Fresh Produce Safety," FDA Talk Paper, May 26, 2000, available at http://cfsan.fda.gov/~lrd/tpproduc.html.

45. Robert V. Tauxe, "Egg-Associated *Salmonella* Enteritidis Infections," speech given before Food and Drug Administration/U.S. Department of Agriculture, Joint Public Meeting, Washington, D.C., September 15, 1998.

46. Ibid.; *Salmonella* Enteritidis Risk Assessment Team, "*Salmonella* Enteritidis Risk Assessment—Shell Eggs and Egg Products," prepared for the Food Safety and Inspection Service, rev. August 10, 1998, available at www.fsis.usda.gov/ophs/risk/index.htm.

47. "Egg Industry Statement Regarding Egg Safety," press statement, Aronow & Pollock Communications, Washington, D.C., June 29, 1999.

48. "Outbreak of Salmonellosis Associated with Eating at Restaurant A, Henrico County, May–June 1999." Unpublished case study by Henrico County.

49. Smith DeWaal et al., *Outbreak Alert!,* pp. 26–31; Elizabeth Dahl and Caroline Smith DeWaal, *Scrambled Eggs* (Washington, D.C.: Center for Science in the Public Interest, 1997), p. 3; European Commission, "Opinion of the Scientific Committee on Veterinary Measures Relating to Public Health on Foodborne Zoonoses," Health and Consumer Protection Directorate-General (April 12, 2000).

50. Food and Drug Administration, *Grade "A" Pasteurized Milk Ordinance,* 1993 Revision, Public Health Service/Food and Drug Administration Publication no. 229, available at www.cfsan.fda.gov/~ear/pmo-1993.html.

51. University of Guelph Dairy Science and Technology, "Pasteurization," available at www.foodsci.uoguelph.ca/dairyedu/pasteurization.html.

52. Barbara Mahon et al., "Consequences in Georgia of a Nationwide Outbreak of *Salmonella* Infections: What You Don't Know Might Hurt You," *American Journal of Public Health* 89 (1999), pp. 31–35.

53. Food and Drug Administration, *Grade "A" Pasteurized Milk Ordinance,*

1999 Revision, Public Health Service/ Food and Drug Administration Publication no. 229, p. v; Food and Drug Administration, Final Rule, "Requirements Affecting Raw Milk for Human Consumption in Interstate Commerce," *Federal Register* 52, no. 153 (August 10, 1987), p. 29509.

54. Bureau of National Affairs, "Listeria Crisis Grips Cheese Industry; Government to Reassure Consumers," *International News* 1, no. 12 (1999), p. 346; Sara H. Cody et al., "Two Outbreaks of Multidrug-Resistant *Salmonella* Serotype Typhimurium DT104 Infections Linked to Raw-Milk Cheese in Northern California," *Journal of the American Medical Association* 281, no. 19 (May 19, 1999), pp. 1805–1810.

55. Food and Drug Administration, *Grade "A" Pasteurized Milk Ordinance;* Michael J. Linnan et al., "Epidemic Listeriosis Associated with Mexican-Style Cheese," *New England Journal of Medicine* 319, no. 13 (1988), pp. 823–828.

56. Linnan et al., "Epidemic Listeriosis"; Elliot T. Ryser and Elmer H. Marth, eds., *Listeria, Listeriosis, and Food Safety* (New York: Marcel Dekker, 1999), pp. 309–316.

57. Betty Harden, Retail Food and Interstate Travel Team, Letter on Aged Hard Cheeses, U.S. Food and Drug Administration, Center for Food Safety and Applied Nutrition, April 5, 1999, available at http://vm.cfsan.fda.gov/~ear/rflhrdch.html.

58. Food and Drug Administration, "Procedures for the Safe and Sanitary Processing and Importing of Fish and Fishery Products," *Federal Register* 60, no. 242 (December 18, 1995), pp. 65096–65097.

59. Smith DeWaal et al., *Outbreak Alert!,* pp. 17–21.

60. Paula Kurtzweil, "Critical Steps Toward Safer Seafood," *FDA Consumer* November/December 1997; rev. February 1998 and 1999), p. 1; Cheryl W. Thompson and Amy Goldstein, "Spoiled Fish Sickens 26 World Bank Employees: 'Scombroid Poisoning' Caused by Blue Marlin Served in Cafeteria at DC Headquarters," *Washington Post,* May 31, 1997, pp. B1, B5.

61. Food and Drug Administration, Office of Seafood, "Shellfish-Related *Vibrio vulnificus* Cases/Deaths, 2000," correspondence to Center for Science in the Public Interest.

62. William R. Archer III, Texas Commissioner of Health, News Release from the Texas Department of Health, October 2, 1998; Seema Mehta, "Invading Species Hit State and Nation Hard," *Los Angeles Times,* December 18, 2000.

63. Centers for Disease Control and Prevention, "Viral Gastroenteritis Associated with Eating Oysters—Louisiana, December 1996–January 1997," *Morbidity and Mortality Weekly Reports* 46, no. 47 (November 28, 1997), pp. 1109–1112.

64. Institute of Medicine, *Seafood Safety* (Washington, D.C.: National Academy Press, 1991), p. 320; Charlotte Christin et al. *Death on the Half Shell: The Failure of Regulators and the Shellfish Industry to Prevent Deaths and Illnesses from Gulf Coast Shellfish* (Washington, D.C.: Center for Science in the Public Interest, June 2001).

65. Food and Drug Administration, "Performance Standards for *Vibrio vulnificus:* Request for Comments," *Federal Register* 64, no. 13 (January 21, 1999), p. 3300.

66. Institute of Medicine, *Seafood Safety,* p. 89.

67. "Scombrotoxic Fish Poisoning in New Mexico," *Lancet,* October 1, 1988, p. 808; Jason D. Morrow, M.D., et al., "Evidence That Histamine Is the Causative Toxin of Scombroid-Fish Poisoning," *New England Journal of Medicine* 324, no. 11 (March 14, 1991), p. 717; Jonathan A. Edlow, M.D., "Something Fishy: How the Doctors' Luncheon Sent Epidemiologists Off on a Fishing Expedition," *Boston* magazine (June 1989), pp. 65–66; Brian W. Christman, M.D., correspondence, *New England Journal of Medicine* 325, no. 1 (August 15, 1991), p. 515; Institute of Medicine, *Seafood Safety,* pp. 93–96.

68. Institute of Medicine, National Research Council, *Ensuring Safe Food from Production to Consumption* (Washington, D.C.: National Academy Press, 1998), p. 12.

69. Centers for Disease Control and Prevention, "Biological and Chemical Terrorism: Strategic Plan for Preparedness and Response: Recommendations of the CDC Strategic Planning Workgroup," *Morbidity and Mortality Weekly Report Recommendations and Reports* 49 (RR04) (April 21, 2000), pp. 5–6; John C. Bailar III, "Ensuring Safe Food: An Organizational Perspective," in Scott P. Layne et al., *Firepower in the Lab: Automation in the Fight Against Infectious Diseases and Bioterrorism* (Washington, D.C.: Joseph Henry Press, 2000), p. 139; T. J. Torok et al., "A Large Community Outbreak of Salmonellosis Caused by Intentional Contamination of Restaurant Salad Bars," *Journal of the American Medical Association* (August 6, 1997), pp. 389–395.

70. Bailar, "Ensuring Safe Food," p. 141.

Chapter Three. Eating for the Environment

1. Michael Brower and Warren Leon, *The Consumer's Guide to Effective Environmental Choices: Practical Advice from the Union of Concerned Scientists* (New York: Three Rivers Press, 1999). See this book for an extended discussion of the research methodology and for detailed findings.

2. National Agricultural Statistics Service, *USDA Historical Track Records* (Washington, D.C.: Department of Agriculture, 2001), available at www.usda.gov/nass/pubs/histdata.htm.

3. Robert Howarth et al., *Nutrient Pollution of Coastal Rivers, Bays, and Seas* (Washington, D.C.: Ecological Society of America, 2000), p. 3; David Tilman et al., "Forecasting Agriculturally Driven Global Environmental Change," *Science* (April 13, 2001), p. 281.

4. Merritt Frey et al., *Spilling Swill: A Survey of Factory Farm Water Pollution in 1999* (Washington, D.C.: Clean Water Network and the Izaak Walton League of America, 1999), p. 1; Esther M. Bauer, "Pigging Out in Texas," *Boston Globe,* November 14, 1999.

5. Frey et al., *Spilling Swill,* p. 4. Clean Water and the Izaak Walton League documented over 100 "spills and dumping of manure and other waste products" in 10 states they surveyed (Frey, *Spilling Swill,* p. 1), but a few other states also have large-scale livestock operations and spills. See also Robbin Marks and Rebecca Knuffke, *America's Animal Factories: How States Fail to Prevent Pollution from Livestock Waste* (Washington, D.C.: Clean Water Network and Natural Resources Defense Council, 1998), p. 1.

6. Mercedes Lee et al., *Seafood Lover's Almanac* (Islip, N.Y.: National Audubon Society's Living Oceans Program, 2000), p. 112.

7. Please note that the quantitative analysis in *The Consumer's Guide* was based on the best available data, but not all that data is highly accurate. Any particular number in the results represents an approximation. Nevertheless, the overall patterns are sufficiently clear that we can be confident about food's overall role in environmental damage.

8. The graph is based on the results in Brower and Leon, *Consumer's Guide,* which used 1994 prices—the average price of ground chuck was $1.84 per pound, the average price of chicken was $1.48 per pound (boneless equivalent), and the average price of rice was $0.53 per pound. In that book, we compared a pound of chicken and a pound of hamburger with 1.4 pounds of pasta because they all have the same number of calories, but upon further reflection it doesn't seem appropriate to give extra credit to the beef and chicken just because their fat content drives up the number of calories. So here we compare equal weights of rice, chicken, and beef, but acknowledge that the hamburger and chicken include more protein than the rice. On the other hand, although we don't have data on a high-protein legume like soybeans, we have no reason to believe that their environmental impacts would be very different from rice or pasta.

9. The table below uses pasta as the standard and compares it with rice, chicken, and hamburger.

	Green-house gases	Common air pollution	Toxic air pollution	Common water pollution	Toxic water pollution	Water use	Land use
Hamburger	4.7	3.0	2.7	24.6	6.3	6.8	27.9
Chicken	2.0	2.0	1.7	17.6	2.5	2.3	2.5
Rice	0.9	1.0	0.7	1.4	1.2	2.1	1.7
Pasta	1.0	1.0	1.0	1.0	1.0	1.0	1.0

10. Peter T. Kilborn, "Storm Highlights Flaws in Farm Law in North Carolina," *New York Times,* October 17, 1999; Phil Bowie, "No Act of God," *Amicus Journal* (Winter 2000), p. 18; North Carolina Department of Environment and Natural Resources, *Framework for the Conversion of Anaerobic Swine Waste Lagoons and Sprayfields* (Raleigh: North Carolina Department of Environment and Natural Resources, 1999), p. 2. For a good analysis of the science and economics of large hog farms, their waste-management techniques, and their environmental impacts, see Kathryn Cochran et al., *Dollars and Sense: An Economic Analysis of Alternative Hog Waste Management Technologies* (Washington, D.C.: Environmental Defense, 2000).

11. Cochran, *Dollars and Sense,* p. 12.

12. Environmental Defense Fund, *Hog Lagoons: Pitting Pork Waste Against Public Health and Environment* (Raleigh, N.C.: Environmental Defense Fund, 1999).

13. Cochran, *Dollars and Sense,* p. viii.

14. For these and other policy recommendations related to hogs, see Environmental Defense Fund, *Hog Lagoons,* pp. 9–12; Frey et al., *Spilling Swill,* p. 19; North Carolina Department, *Framework,* passim; Cochran, *Dollars and Sense,* passim; and Marks and Knuffke, *America's Animal Factories,* pp. 145–149.

15. James E. Horne and Maura McDermott, *The Next Green Revolution: Essential Steps to a Healthy, Sustainable Agriculture* (New York: Food Products Press, 2001), pp. 86–87.

16. Bureau of Land Management, *Public Land Statistics, 2000* (Washington, D.C.: Bureau of Land Management, 2001), p. 31. Land rated mid-seral is considered to be in fair condition and accounts for 36 percent of the total. Land rated early-seral is considered to be in poor condition and accounts for 12 percent of the total.

17. Ronnie Ann Cohen and Jennifer Curtis, *Agricultural Solutions: Improving Water Quality in California Through Water Conservation and Pesticide Reduction* (New York: Natural Resources Defense Council, 1998), pp. 9–10.

18. For a solid, accessible overview of sustainable agriculture practices, see Horne and McDermott, *The Next Green Revolution.*

19. John P. Reaganold et al., "Sustainable Agriculture," *Scientific American* (June 1990), p. 112; Horne and McDermott, *The Next Green Revolution,* p. 69.

20. Mark Lipson, *Searching for the "O-Word": An Analysis of the USDA Current Research Information System (CRIS) for Pertinence to Organic Farming* (Santa Cruz, Calif.: Organic Farming Research Foundation, 1997), p. 6.

21. Sean L. Swezey et al., "Comparison of Conventional and Organic Apple Production Systems During Three Years of Conversion to Organic Management in Coastal California," *American Journal of Alternative Agriculture* (November 4, 1998), pp. 162–180; John P. Reganold et al., "Sustainability of Three Apple Production Systems," *Nature* (April 19, 2001), pp. 926–929. For background on the economics and productivity of organic apple production, see David Ganatstein and Patty Dauer, *Trends in Organic Tree Fruit Production in Washington State* (Wenatchee, Wash.: Center for Sustaining Agriculture and Natural Resources, 2000).

22. Cass Petersen et al., *The Rodale Institute Farming Systems Trial: The First 15 Years* (Kutztown, Pa.: Rodale Institute, 1999), p. 1.

23. Daniel Sellen et al., "A Comparison of Financial Returns During Early Transition from Conventional to Organic Vegetable Production," *Journal of Vegetable Crop Production* 1 (1995) 11–39; A. Fliebbach et. al, *Results from a 21-Year-Old Field Trial* (Frick, Switz.: FiBL, 2000). For an early survey of many of the studies comparing the economics and output of organic and conventional farms, see Molly D. Anderson, "Economics of Organic and Low-Input Farming in the United States of America," in N. H. Lampkin and S. Padel, eds., *The Economics of Organic Farming: An International Perspective* (New York: CAB International, 1994), pp. 161–184.

24. Quoted in Barnaby J. Feder, "Organic Farming: Seeking the Mainstream," *New York Times,* April 9, 2000.

25. Ibid.

26. Ron Scherer, "Farm-Fresh in the City," *Christian Science Monitor,* August 29, 2001.

27. United Nations Development Programme (UNDP) et al., *World Resources, 2000–2001* (Washington, D.C.: World Resources Institute, 2000), p. 70; Food and Agriculture Organization (FAO), *The State of World Fisheries and Aquaculture, 2000* (Rome: Food and Agriculture Organization), pt. 1, p. 11; National Marine Fisheries Service, *Our Living Oceans: Report on the Status of U.S. Living Marine Resources, 1999* (Washington, D.C.: Department of Commerce, 1999), p. 2.

28. World Wildlife Fund, *The Status of Wild Atlantic Salmon: A River by River*

Assessment (Washington, D.C.: World Wildlife Fund, 2001), p 83.; Tracy Basile, "Swordfish Surprise," *Amicus Journal* (Winter 2001), p. 44.

29. Quoted in Michael Harris, *Lament for an Ocean: The Collapse of the Atlantic Cod Fishery: A True Crime Story* (Toronto: McClelland and Stewart, 1998), p. 43. Harris's book unravels the causes behind the Grand Banks' collapse. See also Colin Woodard, *Ocean's End: Travels Through the Endangered Seas* (New York: Basic Books, 2000), pp. 57–95.

30. For a good description of the trawlers and their impact, see Harris, *Lament for an Ocean,* pp. 53–61.

31. Colin Woodard, "A Run on the Banks: How Factory Farms Decimated Newfoundland Cod," *Amicus Journal* (March/April 2001), p. 38.

32. Garrett Hardin, "Tragedy of the Commons," *Science* 162 (1968), pp.1243–1248.

33. UNDP, *World Resources, 2000–2001,* p. 78.

34. Lisa Fuss, "State Completes Marine Reserve Plan," *Miami Herald,* April 25, 2001; Robert Wagner, "Abstract: Using Past Marine Reserve Performance as a Guide for Effective Design," *Proceedings of the Annual Meeting of the American Association for the Advancement of Science* (February 2001), pp. 1–12. For a thorough assessment of ecological reserves and how to set up effective ones, see National Research Council, *Marine Protected Areas: Tools for Sustaining Ocean Ecoystems* (Washington, D.C.: National Academy Press, 2001).

35. Quoted in Francis X. Clines, "Warnings Don't Sway Watermen's Faith in the Blue Crab," *New York Times,* May 13, 2001.

36. UNDP, *World Resources, 2000–2001,* p. 76.

37. Ibid.

38. A team of scientists recently documented this trend and showed that it was taking place on a wide scale. See Daniel Pauly et al., "Fishing Down Marine Food Webs," *Science* (February 6, 1998), pp. 860–863.

39. Harris, *Lament for an Ocean,* pp. 74–75; Rosamond L. Naylor et al., "Effect of Aquaculture on World Fish Supplies," *Nature* (June 29, 2000), p. 1021.

40. Naylor et al., "Effect of Aquaculture," pp. 1018–1019; George W. Chamberlain and Stuart M. Barlow, "Fishmeal," a statement in response to "Effect of Aquaculture on World Fish Supplies," Global Aquaculture Alliance website, available at www.gaalliance.org, 2000.

41. FAO, *World Fisheries,* p. 5.

42. Mary Anne Clancy, "100,000 Salmon Escape from Pens," *Bangor Daily News,* February 23, 2001; Standing Senate Committee on Fisheries, *Aquaculture in Canada's Atlantic and Pacific Regions: Interim Report* (Ottawa, Ont: Standing Senate Committee on Fisheries, 2001).

43. Stuart Miller, "How the King of Fish Is Being Farmed to Death," *Observer,* January 7, 2001.

44. For an overview of the concerns raised about shrimp farming, see Claude E. Boyd and Jason W. Clay, "Shrimp Aquaculture and the Environment," *Scientific American* (June 1998), pp. 58–65. For a more anti-shrimp-farming perspective, see the materials from the Mangrove Action Project on the website of the Earth Island Institute, available at www.earthisland.org/map.

45. Peter Auster, statement at a press conference announcing a special issue of *Conservation Biology,* December 14, 1998, available at www.american oceans.org.

46. Ibid.

47. L. Watling and Elliott A. Norse, "Disturbance of the Seabed by Mobile Fishing Gear: A Comparison to Forest Clear-Cutting," *Conservation Biology* (December 1998), pp. 1180–1197.

48. Les Watling, statement at a press conference announcing a special issue of *Conservation Biology,* December 14, 1998, available at www.americanoceans.org.

49. See www.environmentaldefense.org; www.audubon.org; www.mbayaq.org; and www.nrdc.org. The Seafood Choices Alliance (www.seafoodchoices.org) has a database that includes the recommendations from all of these groups.

50. Lee, *Seafood Lover's Almanac.*

51. Mark Kurlansky, transcript of interview for the PBS television program *Empty Oceans, Empty Nets,* 1999, available at www.habitatmedia.org.

Chapter Four. Pesticides and Chemicals in the Food Supply

1. Environmental Protection Agency, Office of Policy Analysis, *Unfinished Business: A Comparative Assessment of Environmental Problems,* vol. 1, February 1987, p. 84.

2. Center for Science in the Public Interest, "Poll Shows Broad but Limited Support for Labeling of Bioengineered Foods," May 16, 2001, news release, available at www.cspinet.org/new/labeling_gefoods.html.

3. Philip Shabecoff, "Hazard Reported in Apple Chemical," *New York Times,* February 2, 1989, p. A1; Winston Williams, "Polishing the Apple's Image," *New York Times,* May 25, 1986, p. C4; Kenneth Smith and Jack Raso, M.S., R.D., *An Unhappy Anniversary: The Alar "Scare" Ten Years Later* (New York: American Council on Science and Health, 1999); "Correction to 'Personal Health; Health Scares That Weren't So Scary,' " *New York Times,* August 18, 1998; Environmental Working Group, "Ten Years Later, Myth of

'Alar Scare' Persists: How the Chemical Industry Rewrote the History of a Banned Pesticide," February 1999, available at www.ewg.org/reports/alar/alar.html; Consumer's Union, "Alar Shifts the Focus of Public Debate," excerpt from "Pest Management at the Crossroads," 1996, available at www.ecologic-ipm.com/pmac_alar.html.

4. Smith and Raso, *An Unhappy Anniversary,* p. 2.

5. Williams, "Polishing the Apple's Image," p. C4.

6. Michael F. Jacobson, Ph.D., et al., *Funding Safer Farming* (Washington, D.C.: Center for Science in the Public Interest, 1995), p. 1–2; David Pimentel et. al., *Techniques for Reducing Pesticide Use* (Chichester, U.K.: John Wiley & Sons, 1997), p. 1.

7. Arnold L. Aspelin, Ph.D., and Arthur H. Grube, Ph.D., Office of Pesticide Programs, *Pesticides Industry Sales and Usage: 1996 and 1997 Market Estimates* (Washington, D.C.: Environmental Protection Agency), p. 3

8. Ibid., Table 6; National Research Council, *Pesticides in the Diets of Infants and Children* (Washington, D.C.: National Academy Press, 1993), p. 342; Bala Wong, *Play at Your Own Risk: The Hidden Dangers of Pesticide Use in Texas City Parks* (Texas Pesticide Information Network, Consumers Union Southwest Regional Office Report, March 2001), p. 12.

9. Jacobson et al., *Funding Safer Farming,* p. 5.

10. Ibid.

11. Pimentel et al., *Techniques for Reducing Pesticide Use,* p. 4.

12. James E. Horne and Maura McDermott, *The Next Green Revolution: Essential Steps to a Healthy, Sustainable Agriculture* (New York: Food Products Press, 2001), p. 189.

13. Aspelin and Grube, *Pesticide Industry Sales and Usage: 1996 and 1997 Market Estimates,* p. 4; Allen Rosenfeld et al., *Agrichemicals in America: Farmers' Reliance on Pesticides and Fertilizers* (Washington, D.C.: Public Voice for Food and Health Policy, May 1993), p. 24; Robert L. Kellogg, Margaret S. Maizel, and Don W. Goss, *Agricultural Chemical Use and Groundwater Quality: Where Are the Potential Problem Areas?* (Washington, D.C.: Department of Agriculture, 1992), p. A-6; *State of the Environment: A View Toward the Nineties* (Washington, D.C.: Conservation Foundation, 1987), p. 352.

14. Rosenfeld et al., *Agrichemicals in America,* pp. 2, 4.

15. Food and Drug Administration, Center for Food Safety and Applied Nutrition, *Food and Drug Administration Pesticide Program: Residue Monitoring, 1999* (Washington, D.C.: Food and Drug Administration, April 2000), p. 10, available at www.cfsan.fda.gov/~acrobat/pes99rep.pdf.

16. *Food Safety: Overview of Federal and State Expenditures* (Washington,

D.C.: General Accounting Office, 2001), p. 4; Michael F. Jacobson, Ph.D., and Bruce Maxwell, *What Are We Feeding Our Kids?* (New York: Workman Publishing, 1994), p. 77.

17. Multiple chemical sensitivity is a set of illnesses caused by exposure to more than one chemical at significantly lower exposure levels than would result in noticeable illness in the general population.

18. Jennifer Curtis, Tim Profeta, and Lawrie Mott, *After Silent Spring: The Unsolved Problems of Pesticide Use in the United States* (Washington, D.C.: Natural Resources Defense Council, 1993), p. 4.

19. Ibid., p. 9; Robert Repetto and Sanjay S. Baliga, *Pesticides and the Immune System: The Public Health Risks* (Washington, D.C.: World Resources Institute, March 1996), pp. 41–43.

20. Jacobson et al., *Funding Safer Farming,* p. 5.

21. Bruce S. Wilson, "Appendix A: Legislative History of the Pesticide Residues Amendment of 1954 and the Delaney Clause of the Food Additives Amendment of 1958," in National Research Council of the National Academy of Sciences, *Regulating Pesticides in Food: The Delaney Paradox* (Washington, D.C.: National Academy Press, 1987), pp. 161–173.

22. National Research Council, *Regulating Pesticides,* pp. 1–2 .

23. Douglas T. Sheehy, "A *De Minimis* Exception to the Delaney Clause: A Reassessment of *Les v. Reilly,*" *Food and Drug Law Journal* 50 (1995), p. 261; Environmental Working Group, "The Nation's New Pesticide Law," October 1996, available at www.ewg.org/reports/newpestlaw/newpestlaw.html.

24. Curtis, Profeta, and Mott, *After Silent Spring,* pp. 22–23.

25. National Research Council, *Regulating Pesticides,* pp. 40–41.

26. *Les et al. v. Reilly,* 968 F.2d 985 (9th Cir. 1992), *cert. denied,* 507 U.S. 950 (1993).

27. Ibid.

28. National Research Council, *Pesticides in the Diets of Infants and Children,* p. 2.

29. Ibid.

30. Consumers Union, *A Report Card for the EPA: Successes and Failures in Implementing the Food Quality Protection Act,* February 2001, pp. 3, 4; pt. 3, p. 5.

31. Todd Hettenbach and Richard Wiles. *Attack of the Killer Weeds: Pesticide Hypocrisy on Capitol Hill* (Washington, D.C.: Environmental Working Group, 1999), pp. ii, 17.

32. Ibid., p. 18.

33. Peter Orris et al., *Persistent Organic Pollutants and Human Health* (N.p.: World Federation of Public Health Associations, May 2000); Theo Colborn, Dianne Dumanoski, and John Peterson Myers, *Our Stolen Future: Are We*

Threatening Our Fertility, Intelligence, and Survival? A Scientific Detective Story (New York: Penguin Group, 1996).

34. "Produce Safety: New Data on Pesticide Levels," *Consumer Reports Online* (September 2000), available at www.consumerreports.org.

35. Erik D. Olson, "Testimony on the Implementation of the Safe Drinking Water Act Amendments of 1996," October 8, 1998, citing J. V. Bennet et al., "Infectious and Parasitic Diseases," in R. Ambler and H. B. Dull, eds., *Closing the Gap: The Burden of Unnecessary Illness* (New York: Oxford University Press, 1987); Michael Kramer et al., "Surveillance for Waterborne-Disease Outbreaks—United States, 1993-1994," *CDC Morbidity and Mortality Weekly Report Surveillance Summaries* 45, no. 55-1 (April 12, 1996), p. 1; "Fact Sheets: *Cryptosporidium,*" American Water Works Association, rev. February 18, 2000, available at www.awwa.org/pressroom/crypto.htm.

36. U.S. Geological Survey, "Ground Water Studies," August 16, 1995, available at www.water.usgs.gov/wid/html/GW.html.; Environmental Protection Agency, *National Water Quality Inventory, 1998 Report to Congress, Ground Water and Drinking Water Chapters* (Washington, D.C.: Environmental Protection Agency, 1998) pp. 13–14, available at www.epa.gov/safewater/protect/98_305b_all.pdf.

37. National Research Council, *Alternative Agriculture* (Washington, D.C.: National Academy Press, 1989), p. 54; Thomas C. Winter et al., *Ground Water and Surface Water: A Single Resource,* U.S. Geological Survey Circular 1139 (Denver: U.S. Geological Survey, 1998), p. 64.

38. Barry Brown, "Ontario Medical Officer Questions Safety of Deep-Well Water After *E. Coli* Deaths," *Buffalo News,* October 15, 2000, p. 3A; National Research Council, *Alternative Agriculture,* p. 99; Winter et al., *Ground Water;* Environmental Protection Agency, Office of Water, "Current Drinking Water Standards," updated September 7, 2001, available at www.epa.gov/safewater/ mcl.html.

39. World Health Organization, fact sheet no. 210, "Arsenic in Drinking Water," rev. May 2001, available at www.who.int/inf-fs/en/fact210.html.

40. Subcommittee on Arsenic in Drinking Water, National Research Council, National Academy of Sciences, *Arsenic in Drinking Water* (Washington, D.C.: National Academy Press, 1999), p. 301.

41. Natural Resources Defense Council, press release, "NRDC Denounces Bush Administration Suspension of Arsenic-in-Drinking-Water Protections," May 22, 2001. The reason there is a push worldwide to go under 10 ppb is because there is an increased cancer risk at concentrations above 10 ppb.

42. Erik Olson, "Safe Drinking Water Act Amendments of 1996: Section-by-

Section Summary," August 7, 1996, Natural Resources Defense Council, available at www.nrdc.org/water/drinking/asdwa96.asp.

43. Colborn, Dumanoski, and Myers, *Our Stolen Future,* p. 24.

44. Thomas Stuttaford, "Perils of Mercury," *Times* (London), March 22, 2001.

45. Trade Environment Database Case Studies, case no. 246, "Minamata Disaster," American University, January 11, 1997, available at www.american.edu/ted/minamata.htm; "Fact Sheet: Mercury Update: Impact on Fish Advisories," Environmental Protection Agency, Office of Water, September 20, 1999.

46. Institute of Medicine, *Seafood Safety,* pp. 116–117, 162.

47. See "Listing of Fish and Wildlife Advisories," available at http://fish.rti.org. This site has links to local, state, and federal advisories.

48. Centers for Disease Control and Prevention, "Blood and Hair Mercury Levels in Young Children and Women of Childbearing Age—United States, 1999," *CDC Morbidity and Mortality Weekly Report* 50, no. 8 (March 2, 2001), pp.140–143.

49. Center for Science in the Public Interest, "Throw Back the Fish," *Nutrition Action Healthletter* 28, no. 7 (September 2001), p. 8.

50. 15 U.S.C. § 2605; 21 CFR § 109.15.

51. Kristin Schafer et al., *Nowhere to Hide: Persistent Toxic Chemicals in the U.S. Food Supply* (San Francisco: Pesticide Action Network North American and Commonweal, 2000), p. 23.

52. "Paternal Concentrations of Dioxin and Sex Ratio of Offspring," *Lancet,* May 27, 2000, pp. 1858–1863.

53. Institute of Medicine, Committee to Review the Health Effects in Vietnam Veterans of Exposure to Herbicides, *Veterans and Agent Orange, Update 1998* (Washington, D.C.: National Academy Press, 1999); Department of Veterans Affairs, news release "VA Links Agent Orange and Diabetes," November 9, 2000.

54. Colborn, Dumanoski, and Myers, *Our Stolen Future,* pp. 190–191; Jim Barlow, "Heavy Consumption of Tainted Fish Curbs Adult Learning and Memory," *U Ideas of General Interest,* University of Illinois at Urbana-Champaign, June 2001, available at www.newswise.com/articles/2001/6/pcbfish.uil.html.

55. World Health Organization, "Questions and Answers About Dioxins and Their Effects on Human Health," July 9, 1999; Center for Science in the Public Interest, "Dioxin for Dinner," *Nutrition Action Healthletter* (October 2000), pp. 3, 7.

56. Center for Science in the Public Interest, "Dioxin for Dinner," pp. 3, 7.

57. Ibid., p. 4.

Chapter Five. Ten Steps to a Healthy Diet

1. Department of Agriculture, Agricultural Research Service, *Results from USDA's 1994–96 Diet and Health Knowledge Survey, Table Set 19* (Beltsville, Md.: Department of Agriculture, 2000), pp. 20, 36, 42, 43, 48, 62; Department of Agriculture, Agricultural Research Service, *Pyramid Servings Data: Results from USDA's 1994-96 Continuing Survey of Food Intakes by Individuals, Table Set 9* (Beltsville, Md.: Department of Agriculture, 1999), p. 9.

2. Department of Agriculture, Economic Research Service, "Briefing Room: Diet and Health: Food Consumption and Nutrient Intake Tables," nutrient intake Table 2, available at www.ers.usda.gov/briefing/DietAndHealth/data.

3. Bonnie Liebman, "Defensive Eating: Staying Lean in a Fattening World," *Nutrition Action Healthletter* (December 2001), p. 1.

4. Brownell quoted in ibid. For a discussion of public policies the government could implement to promote better nutrition and health, see Marion Nestle and Michael Jacobson, "Halting the Obesity Epidemic: A Public Health Policy Approach," *Public Health Report* (January/February 2000).

5. J. Michael McGinnis and William F. Foege, "Actual Causes of Death in the United States," *Journal of the American Medical Association* (November 10, 1993), p. 2208; Francisco Fuentes et al., "Mediterranean and Low-Fat Diets Improve Endothelial Function in Hypocholesterolemic Men," *Annals of Internal Medicine* (June 19, 2001), pp. 1115–1119.

6. Bonnie Liebman, "Diseases We Can Prevent," *Nutrition Action Healthletter* (December 1999), p. 5.

7. Liebman and Schardt, "Diet and Health," p. 6.

8. Anthony DeBarros, "Fast-Food Highway Hazards," *USA Today,* June 1, 2001.

9. Liebman and Schardt, "Diet and Health," pp. 6–7.

10. "Cake on Steroids," *Nutrition Action Healthletter* (June 2001), p. 16.

11. Bonnie Liebman and Jayne Hurley, *Healthy Foods: Your Guide to the Best Basic Foods* (Washington, D.C.: Center for Science in the Public Interest, n.d.), pp. 14–15.

12. Ibid., p. 10.

13. Simin Liu et al., "Intake of Vegetables Rich in Carotenoids and Risk of Coronary Heart Disease in Men," *International Journal of Epidemiology* (February 2001), pp. 130–135.

14. "In the Drink: When It Comes to Calories, Solid Is Better Than Liquid," *Nutrition Action Healthletter* (November 2000), pp. 7-9.

15. Quoted in Bonnie Liebman, "Vitamins and Minerals: How Much Is Too

Much?" *Nutrition Action Healthletter* (June 2001), p. 8. See Liebman's article for a rundown of the potential adverse effects from excessive intake of 20 vitamins and minerals.

Chapter Six. The Farmer's New Genes: The Safety of Biotechnology

1. Heather Scoffield, "Canola Farmer Fights Seed Invasion," *Toronto Globe and Mail,* August 14, 2000.

2. Donna U. Vogt and Mickey Parish, *Food Biotechnology in the United States: Science, Regulation, and Issues* (Washington, D.C.: Congressional Research Service, 1999), p. 3.

3. Alan McHughen, *Pandora's Picnic Basket: The Potential and Hazards of Genetically Modified Foods* (New York: Oxford University Press, 2000), pp. 47–48.

4. David Barboza, "U.S. Farmers Still Planting Biotech Crops," *New York Times,* July 1, 2000; "Agricultural Biotechnology," *Nature Biotechnology* (June 1999), p. 612.

5. Royal Society of London et al., *Transgenic Plants and World Agriculture* (Washington, D.C.: National Academy Press, 2000).

6. Claire Cockeroft, "Yielding Results," *Guardian* (U.K.), June 14, 2001.

7. Craig S. Smith, "China Rushes to Adopt Genetically Modified Crops," *New York Times,* October 7, 2000; Carl Pray et al., "Impact of Bt Cotton in China," *World Development* (May 2001), pp. 813–825.

8. David E. Ervin et al., *Transgenic Crops: An Environmental Assessment* (Arlington, Va.: Henry A. Wallace Center for Agricultural and Environmental Policy, 2000); Leonard P. Gianessi and Cressida S. Silvers, "The Potential for Biotechnology to Improve Crop Pest Management in the U.S.: 30-Crop Study," preliminary results presented at BIO 2001, San Diego, Calif., June 25, 2001, pp. 8, 13; Janet E. Carpenter, *Case Studies in Benefits and Risks of Agricultural Biotechnology: Roundup Ready Soybeans and Bt Field Corn* (Washington, D.C.: National Center for Food and Agricultural Policy, 2001), p. 1.

9. Carpenter, *Case Studies,* passim.

10. Gordon Conway, "Genetically Modified Crops: Risks and Promises," *Conservation and Ecology* (June 2000), available online at www.consecol.org/Journal.; Brian Larkins, comments at the Workshop to Assess the Regulatory Oversight of GM Crops and the Next Generation of Genetic Modification for Crop Plants, National Research Council, October 13, 2000.

11. Conway, "Genetically Modified Crops."

12. Adamu quoted in "How Will We Feed Ourselves?" *AgBiotech Bulletin* (November 2000), p. 1; United Nations Development Programme, *Human De-*

velopment Report, 2001: Making New Technologies Work for Human Development (New York: Oxford University Press, 2001), p. 35.

13. Patrick A. Nielson, letter to the Subcommittee on Environmental Impacts Associated with Commercialization of Transgenic Crops of the National Research Council, September 5, 2000.

14. Alan McHughen, *Pandora's Picnic Basket: The Potential and Hazards of Genetically Modified Foods* (New York: Oxford University Press, 2000), pp. 193–195.

15. Ibid., pp. 119–120.

16. Jennifer Van Brunt, "The Battle of Engineered Tomatoes," *Bio/Technology* (July 1992), p. 748; Marion Nestle, "Food Biotechnology: Truth in Advertising," *Bio/Technology* (September 1992), p. 1056; Russ Hoyle, "Eating Biotechnology," *Bio/Technology* (June 1992), p. 629; Nestle, "Food Biotechnology," p. 1056. For the complete story of the Flavr Savr tomato, see Brenda Martineau, *First Fruit: The Creation of the Flavr Savr Tomato and the Birth of Biotech Food* (New York: McGraw-Hill, 2001).

17. Vogt and Parish, *Food Biotechnology in the United States,* pp. 7–8.

18. Ortwin Renn, "European Attitudes Towards Biotechnology," paper delivered at the Kennedy School of Government, Harvard University, June 21, 2000; His Royal Highness the Prince of Wales, "Seeds of Disaster," *Ecologist* (September/October 1999), pp. 252–253.

19. Carol Kaesuk Yoon, "E.P.A. Announces New Rules on Genetically Altered Corn," *New York Times,* January 17, 2000.

20. Holliday quoted in David Barboza, "Biotech Companies Take On Critics of Gene-Altered Food," *New York Times,* November 12, 1999; Shapiro quoted in Kurt Eichenwald, "Biotechnology Food: From the Lab to a Debacle," *New York Times,* January 25, 2001.

21. William Claiborne, "Biotech Crops Spur Warning," *Washington Post,* November 24, 1999.

22. Bryan O'Reilly, "Reaping a Biotech Blunder," *Fortune* (February 19, 2001), pp. 156–164.

23. Philip Brasher, "Corn Recall Now Affects Outlets Across the Country," *Austin American-Statesman,* November 3, 2000; Anthony Shadid, "Tests for Genetic Corn Spur Concerns," *Boston Globe,* May 3, 2001.

24. Quoted in Dale Kasler, "Corn Furor Stalls Biotech Drive," *Sacramento Bee,* November 3, 2000.

25. Laurent Belsie, "No Bumper Crop of Genetically Altered Plants," *Christian Science Monitor,* August 30, 2001.

26. ISAAA, press release, "Global GM Crop Area Continues to Grow," January 10, 2002.

27. "U.S. Regulatory System Needs Adjustment as Volume and Mix of Transgenic Plants Increase in Marketplace," press release, National Academy of Sciences, Washington, D.C., April 5, 2000.

28. Jane Rissler and Margaret Mellon, *The Ecological Risks of Engineered Crops* (Cambridge, Mass.: MIT Press, 1996), p. 28. This book includes an extensive discussion of the risk of creating new weeds.

29. David Pimentel, letter to the Subcommittee on Environmental Impacts Associated with Commercialization of Transgenic Crops of the National Research Council, September 2000.

30. The federal government is belatedly beginning to address the invasive species problem. An interagency report, released in 2001, sketched out useful actions that the government should take, but it is too soon to tell how strong or effective the government's actions will be. For the report, see National Invasive Species Council, *Management Plan: Meeting the Invasive Species Challenge* (Washington, D.C.: National Invasive Species Council, 2001), and for updated information on government initiatives, visit www.invasivespecies.gov.

31. Carol Kaesuk Yoon, "Squash with Altered Genes Raises Fears of 'Superweeds,'" *New York Times,* November 3, 1999.

32. Committee on Genetically Modified Pest-Protected Plants, *Genetically Modified Pest-Protected Plants: Science and Regulation* (Washington, D.C.: National Research Council, 2000), p. 125.

33. Anthony Shadid, "Blown Profits," *Boston Globe,* April 8, 2001.

34. Committee on Genetically Modified Pest-Protected Plants, *Pest-Protected Plants,* p. 103. For the early views of ecologists, see Margaret Mellon and Jane Rissler, eds., *Now or Never: Serious New Plans to Save a Natural Pest Control* (Cambridge, Mass.: Union of Concerned Scientists, 1998).

35. Chris Hables Gray, letter to the Subcommittee on Environmental Impacts Associated with Commercialization of Transgenic Crops of the National Research Council, August 30, 2000.

36. For fascinating stories of unexpected impacts from past introduced species, see Kim Todd, *Tinkering with Eden: A Natural History of Exotics in America* (New York: W. W. Norton, 2001).

37. Ervin et al., *Transgenic Crops,* p. 52.

38. Kenneth Mallory and Mark Chandler, *Lake Victoria: Africa's Inland Sea* (Boston: New England Aquarium, 2000), pp. 11–20.

39. Aqua Bounty Farms website, www.webhost.avint.net/afprotein/bounty.htm; W. M. Muir and R. D. Howard, "Possible Ecological Risks of Transgenic Organism Release When Transgenes Affect Mating Success," *Proceedings of the National Academy of Sciences* (November 23, 1999), pp. 13853–13856.

40. Steven Fondriest, "Sliced Salmon on Rye," *Nucleus* (Winter 2000–01), p. 2.

41. Aqua Bounty Farms website, www.webhost.avint.net/afprotein/bounty.htm. Some critics worry that the technology for producing sterile fish will not always work flawlessly. See, for example, Fondriest, "Sliced Salmon on Rye," p. 2.

42. Goldberg quoted in David L. Chandler, "Down on the Farm," *Boston Globe,* September 26, 2000.

43. Quoted in John Robbins, *The Food Revolution: How Your Diet Can Help Save Your Life and the World* (Berkeley, Calif.: Conari Press, 2001), p. 342.

44. Center for Science in the Public Interest, *National Opinion Poll on Labeling of Genetically Engineered Foods* (Washington, D.C.: Center for Science in the Public Interest, 2001).

45. For an extensive discussion of all the intricacies and complications of labeling by an opponent, see McHughen, *Pandora's Picnic Basket,* pp. 201–229.

46. "The Name of the Game," *New Scientist* (May 22, 1999), p. 3.

Chapter 7. Microwave Ovens, Shade-Grown Coffee, and Other Good Environmental Choices

1. The figures in the chapter and the table below are based on the data collected for Michael Brower and Warren Leon, *The Consumer's Guide to Effective Environmental Choices: Practical Advice from the Union of Concerned Scientists* (New York: Three Rivers Press, 1999). The numbers in this table are somewhat different from the ones reported in that book, because some aspects of food production (especially fertilizers and agricultural chemicals) were mistakenly included in the "Other/Indeterminate" category, rather than under "Cultivation," where they rightly belong. There is still a large "Indeterminate" category because of the limitations of the data.

THE ROLES OF CULTIVATION, PROCESSING, PACKAGING, AND TRANSPORTATION FOR FRUITS, VEGETABLES, AND GRAINS

	Greenhouse gases	Common air pollution	Toxic air pollution	Common water pollution	Toxic water pollution	Water use	Land use
Cultivation	9%	54%	47%	78%	46%	99%	82%
Food processing	20%	6%	1%	4%	8%	0%	1%

	Green-house gases	Common air pollution	Toxic air pollution	Common water pollution	Toxic water pollution	Water use	Land use
Packaging	6%	4%	9%	5%	11%	0%	9%
Transpor-tation	24%	15%	19%	0%	0%	0%	7%
Retail	2%	1%	5%	1%	0%	0%	1%
Other/Inde-terminate	38%	20%	18%	12%	34%	0%	1%

2. Smithsonian Migratory Bird Center, "Why Migratory Birds Are Crazy for Coffee," n.d., available at www.si.edu/smbc.

3. Robert Rice and Justin Ward, *Coffee, Conservation, and Commerce in the Western Hemisphere: How Individuals and Institutions Can Promote Ecologically Sound Farming and Forest Management in Northern Latin America* (Washington, D.C.: Natural Resources Defense Council and Smithsonian Migratory Bird Center, 1996), pp. 3, 10.

4. Ibid., pp. 12–13; Smithsonian Migratory Bird Center, "Why Migratory Birds Are Crazy."

5. Oxfam, *Bitter Coffee: How the Poor Are Paying for the Slump in Coffee Prices* (Oxford, U.K.: Oxfam, 2001), pp. 2, 5, 10.

6. Nick Mathiason and Patrick Tooher, "World Takes Caffeine Hit," *Observer,* August 12, 2001.

7. Tanzanian farmer quoted in Oxfam, *Bitter Coffee,* p. 1; Nicaraguan mother Yamileth Davila quoted in David Gonzalez, "A Coffee Crisis' Devastating Domino Effect in Nicaragua," *New York Times,* August 29, 2001.

8. Quoted in Elizabeth Neuffer, "Cooperative Looks for Bigger Share of the Profits for Growers," *Boston Globe,* July 29, 2001.

9. See Brower and Leon, *Consumer's Guide* for more on this topic.

10. Alex Wilson and John Morrill, *Consumer Guide to Home Energy Savings,* rev. ed. (Washington, D.C.: American Council for an Energy-Efficient Economy, 1996), pp. 191–192.

11. Franklin Associates, *Resource and Environmental Profile Analysis of Polyethylene and Unbleached Paper Grocery Sacks,* report prepared for the Council for Solid Waste Solutions, June 1990.

12. Ibid., pp. 4-8–4-9.

Chapter Eight. Building the Safest Food Supply: A Menu of Actions to Improve Your Community and Influence the Government

1. Institute of Medicine, National Research Council, *Ensuring Safe Food from Production to Consumption* (Washington, D.C.: National Academy Press, 1998), p. 12.

INDEX

Page numbers in *italics* indicate charts and figures.